Patient-Based Medicine

Patient-Based Medicine:

Treat the Patient, Not the Disease

By

Johannes G. Schmidt and

Richard Evan Steele

Cambridge Scholars Publishing

Patient-Based Medicine:
Treat the Patient, Not the Disease

By Johannes G. Schmidt and Richard Evan Steele

This book first published 2023

Cambridge Scholars Publishing

Lady Stephenson Library, Newcastle upon Tyne, NE6 2PA, UK

British Library Cataloguing in Publication Data
A catalogue record for this book is available from the British Library

ISBN (10): 1-5275-4350-1
ISBN (13): 978-1-5275-4350-8

TABLE OF CONTENTS

CHAPTER ONE

THE CONCEPT OF CLINICAL RESEARCH OR THE END OF DISCUSSION ABOUT PLACEBO AND SPECIFIC EFFECTS

Preliminary remark: It started with a thorough analysis
http://www.paracelsus-heute.ch/cms/literatur/011_wiss_einsiedler_symposium/0113.php

The reorientation of clinical research towards the questions of treatment benefit (beyond the question of treatment efficacy) and of how much clinical trials represent actual practice (external validity) is the timely path to clinical research questions of real interest and importance. Postmodern anything goes makes it possible to also consider hitherto dismissed effects, such as placebo, as valuable. However, that would require a precise documentation of the external validity of such effects. Not disease as such, but the disease context, not therapy as such, but the therapeutic context, not the patient as such, but the patient context, not a test as such, but the test situation has become an important focus of clinical research. In respect to test results, current medicine can and should recognize its preoccupation with allegedly objective and hard data. The patient context can determine whether an efficacious therapy is beneficial or harmful. It is thus the proper definition of the patient context which makes medicine documentable, no matter how objective or subjective the effect of therapy is. The consideration of the therapeutic context leads to the important distinction between efficacy and effectiveness (or benefit), and this makes it clear that the randomized controlled trial in its traditional design as the placebo controlled double-blind trial (DBRCT) is limited to the evaluation of drug theory. The evaluation of treatment effectiveness requires more pragmatic trials which study treatment operations and not isolated components and which may also compare entire treatment strategies. Pragmatic clinical trials, in future, will not only allow the study of pathogenesis blockers, but also the study of salutogenic interventions working with the host constitution. The focus of attention and research in the new school of EBM with clinical epidemiology as its basic science, and not mere literature-based medicine, has long ago identified illness as the product of host, disease and environment. Meanwhile, the dispute about placebo and specific effects has become obsolete.

The title of the *3rd Scientific Symposium of Einsiedeln Placebo – Valuable if it Helps the Patient – Methods and Design of a Pragmatic Clinical Research, An orientation towards patient benefit* makes it clear that we will not only discuss speculations about the existence and nature of the placebo effect, but mainly the place of placebo in the context of clinical trials and clinical judgement. The debate as to whether placebo effects exist at all adds to the fact that not every seemingly unexplainable improvement is a placebo effect. The natural course of a disease, sometimes together with a regression to the mean, can lead to improvements, but this rather academic debate is of minor importance for our discussion. Often, placebo is called a non-specific effect. It remains difficult to define what is specific and what is not (see chapters II and III). Placebo is well-defined as a component of the placebo controlled double-blind trial, and its methodological place can be discussed. It is a fact that placebo, which has been disdained as mere conceit and excluded from our clinical thinking, is being rehabilitated.

External validity

With the onset of the age of clinical epidemiology and EBM, a reorientation of clinical research is taking place towards questions of treatment benefit (beyond the question of treatment efficacy) and of how much clinical trials represent actual practice (external validity). This is the timely path to clinical research questions of real interest and importance. Postmodern anything goes makes it possible to consider placebo effects as a valuable part of medicine, not disease as such, but the disease context, not therapy as such, but the therapeutic context, not the patient as such, but the patient context, not a test as such, but the test situation have become important foci of clinical research and critical appraisal of evidence. However, a documentation of the external validity of such effects must be included. What evidence/study result is important for my patient? Sacket et al. put the question everywhere, "*can you apply this [internally] valid, important evidence in caring for your [particular]patient?*" The dogma itself doesn't count, but the precise, empirically verified situation in which the dogma has its validity and results clearly doing more benefit than harm. This change in the understanding of medical science is more revolutionary than it looks and may be as significant as the end of the Middle Ages 500 years ago. It was

Paracelsus that recognized the importance of external validity. He observed that veneration of saints is helpful if it helps to face fear and uncertainty, but that the veneration business run by the church is illusionistic and detrimental to health. The most famous dictum of Paracelsus says: "everything can be venom or cure. The *dose* makes the difference." Dose can also be understood as the context.

Test and test context

Test results in current medicine must take into account that objective and hard data fails to account for spontaneous salutogenesis and the placebo effect. Dismissal of placebo as a medical non-value is based on the belief that modern, conventional medicine cannot take this into account because of the belief that only what is a *hard* and *objective* diagnostic finding is real. This, we tend to reason, makes our method superior to alternative quacks and to the imaginary placebos of earlier times. We will first touch on test and test context and patient and patient context before delving into therapy and therapeutic context. This will then lead into placebo and its place in clinical trials. One can thus elucidate that modern medicine is not necessarily more enlightened than the medicine of earlier times. The pre-test likelihood has the same mathematical power as the technical specificity to influence the post-test likelihood or positive predictive value which is the relevant measure in practice. If the pre-test likelihood is 1 in 100, the false positives will be multiplied by 100 (figure 1). Thus, it is the proper enquiry of the patient history which makes medicine scientific, no matter how objective or subjective the test results may be. If the clinical suspicion of a certain diagnosis is high, then a positive test result means an almost certain confirmation of the diagnosis. If there is no real clinical suspicion as in screenings or in a check-up, a positive result is often false and not much different from the pre-test likelihood. This is the main reason why screenings and check-ups are increasingly viewed as useless as the positive predictive value is not much different from the pre-test likelihood. For example, if there is a high clinical suspicion of coronary heart disease CHD – let us estimate the likelihood to be 1 to 1, a positive result in the exercise ECG will increase the likelihood to 80% (sensitivity is about 70% and specificity 80%) which makes the test rather useful in this situation. If we use the same test in as a check-up in a younger man with no symptoms – let us estimate the likelihood of being 1%. The positive predictive value with the very same result will only be 4%. In more than 95% of cases, the result will be a false positive. The test does not give us useful information. Another example: a negative mammography result in a woman of about 60 years results in a negative predictive value of 99.8%. She is then 99.8% certain that there is no hidden breast cancer that will become apparent in the next 2-3 years. We are happy about this certainty. However, since the incidence is very low, we are already 99.5% certain without mammography that there will be no cancer.

Figure 1.

	Disease				
Test	**True positive**	a	c	**False positive**	Test positive
	False negative	b	d	True negative	Test negative
	Diseased			Healthy	

Sensitivity = a/a+c
Specificity = d/b+d
Positive predictive value (PPD) = a/a+b
Negative predictive value (NPD) = d/c+d
Prevalence = a+b/a+b+c+d

We do not need to apply screening technology to assure us. We do not need to create the risk of false positive results and overdiagnosis. With Paracelsus we can say: futile veneration of saints (in modern clothes). This may show how illiterate and fallacious the ordinary belief is in hard and objective results that leads to modern medicine wrongly believing that we know better than the good doctors did hundreds of years ago.

Patient and the patient context

The patient context determines whether an efficacious therapy is beneficial or harmful, and therefore, it is the proper definition of the patient context which makes medicine scientific, no matter how objective or subjective the effect of a given therapy may be. The existence of a true, confirmed pathological finding does not tell how sick a patient is. The patient context is as much a result of the *base-line risk*. This determines the *number-needed to treat* which is the measure of the absolute risk reduction that can be expected. The very same therapy can be beneficial in a severely diseased person, but harmful in a lightly diseased person. An example: if I treat a woman with severe osteoporosis who has a chance of 50% to suffer a bone fracture within 1 year with a bisphosphonate, which will likely reduce the risk by 50%, she will have a benefit with a chance of 50% or 1:2 respectively. The number needed to treat is only 2 (figure 2). If I treat a healthy woman with no symptoms, but with a low densitometry result which was measured because of the modern densitometry propaganda, the risk is maybe only 2%. It can also be reduced by 50% from 2% to 1%. The number needed to treat is now 100. In the first case the therapy may mean a significant relief, but treatment in the second case will mean possible long-term adverse effects with no clear benefit. The mathematics of the baseline risk and NNT is simple. You have only fully understood the issue when you become aware that the treatment of high blood cholesterol in low-risk persons is less efficient than the treatment of normal blood cholesterol in high-risk persons. The well-known Framingham data illustrate this clearly (figure 3).

Figure 2. Number needed to treat NNT as a function of the extent of risk reduction and the baseline risk.

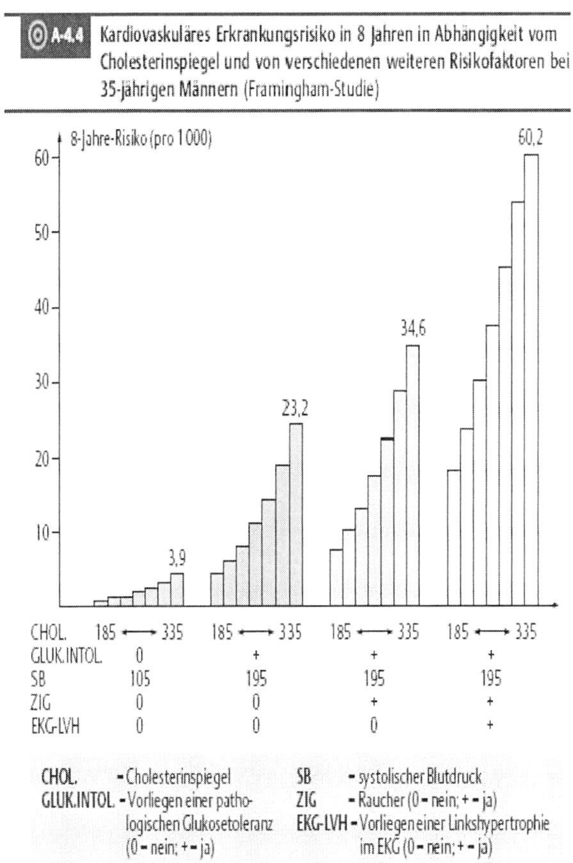

Figure 3. Cardiovascular risk during 8 years depending on multiple risk factors – blood cholesterol, glucose intolerance, systolic hypertension, smoking. Left ventricular hypertrophy. Framingham study 1979.

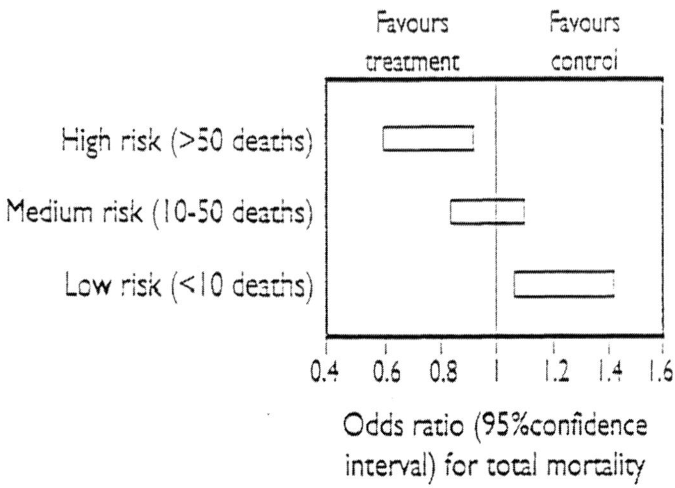

FIG 4—*Effect of cholesterol lowering treatment on total mortality stratified by number of deaths from coronary heart disease per 1000 person years in control subjects*

phy – Framingham study 1979

It is obvious that the risk levels from low to high blood cholesterol are considerably higher if there are risk factors other than blood cholesterol. Lowering blood cholesterol has a greater effect on the risk if the overall risk is high. The notion of normal and pathological cholesterol levels is a fallacy that ignores the probabilistic nature of the risk factor model. The Sheffield Table forms a more adequate approach. They do not assume that there is a cut-off level between normal and pathological cholesterol values, but that we think of persons with elevated risk levels and persons with safe levels that do not require treatment, depending on the overall risk. One could speak of a total risk cut-off level instead of a cholesterol cut-off level. The Sheffield authors chose an arbitrary CHD risk of 3% annually which results in NNT of 100. Persons within these boundaries warrant a regimen of risk factor reduction. Outside the boundaries the total risk is small and the NNT excessively high.

Without a thorough analysis of the context, patients run into the arms of death – led by the race horses of modern medicine. *George Davey Smith* presented his findings on the total mortality effect of cholesterol lowering treatment at the 1st Scientific Symposium of Einsiedeln. He showed that cholesterol lowering treatment increased total mortality in low-risk persons and could only decrease total mortality in high-risk persons (figure 4). Cholesterol lowering treatment reduces mortality to a greater extent than it reduces infarct mortality (Johannes Schmidt. Cholesterol lowering treatment and mortality. Br Med J. 1992:305:1126-1127). It is not surprising that a low total risk and a corresponding high NNT means a cumulation of adverse effects with a possible unintended mortality increase. Cholesterol screening was a bad idea and harmful to many people. Do-gooders can have negative effects in the hands of modern medicine. Alternative practitioners as well as conventional doctors of medicine must use the patient centered parameters to make sure that therapy is beneficial and not harmful.

Figure 4. Effect of cholesterol lowering treatment on total mortality stratified by number of deaths from coronary. heart disease per 1000 person years in control subjects. George Davey Smith. Einsiedeln Symposium, October 1993.

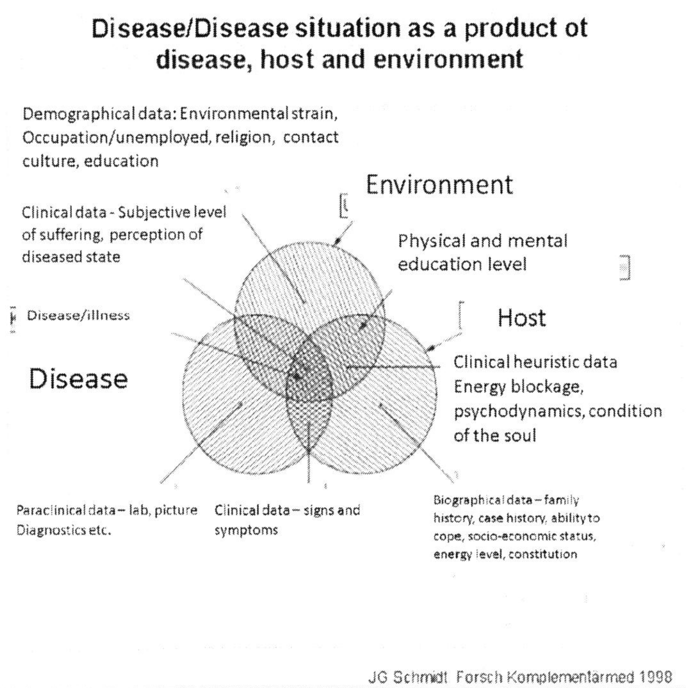

Table 1. Sheffield Table of primary prevention of CHD, The Lancet 1996.

THE LANCET

Men: cholesterol concentration (mmol/L)												
Hypertension	Yes	Yes	Yes	Yes	Yes	No	Yes	Yes	No	No	Yes	No
Smoking	Yes	Yes	No	No	Yes	Yes	Yes	No	Yes	No	No	No
Diabetes	Yes	No	Yes	No	Yes	Yes	No	Yes	No	Yes	No	No
LVH	Yes	Yes	Yes	Yes	No	No	No	No	No	No	No	No
Age (yr)												
70	5·5	5·5	5·5	5·5	5·5	5·5	5·5	5·5	5·5	6·0	6·5	7·7
68	5·5	5·5	5·5	5·5	5·5	5·5	5·5	5·5	5·6	6·4	6·9	8·2
66	5·5	5·5	5·5	5·5	5·5	5·5	5·5	5·7	5·9	6·8	7·3	8·7
64	5·5	5·5	5·5	5·5	5·5	5·5	5·5	6·1	6·3	7·3	7·8	9·3
62	5·5	5·5	5·5	5·5	5·5	5·5	5·6	6·5	6·7	7·8	8·3	
60	5·5	5·5	5·5	5·5	5·5	5·6	6·0	6·9	7·2	8·3	8·9	
58	5·5	5·5	5·5	5·5	5·5	6·1	6·5	7·4	7·7	8·9		
56	5·5	5·5	5·5	5·5	5·5	6·5	7·0	8·0	8·3			
54	5·5	5·5	5·5	5·5	5·9	7·0	7·5	8·6	9·0			
52	5·5	5·5	5·5	5·5	6·3	7·6	8·1	9·3				
50	5·5	5·5	5·5	5·7	6·9	8·2	8·8					
48	5·5	5·5	5·5	6·2	7·5	8·9						
46	5·5	5·5	5·5	6·8	8·2							
44	5·5	5·5	5·8	7·4	9·0							
42	5·5	5·6	6·4	8·2								
40	5·5	6·1	7·1	9·0								
38	5·5	6·8	7·9									
36	6·0	7·6	8·8									
34	6·7	8·6										
32	7·6											
30	8·7											
≤29												

Women: cholesterol concentration (mmol/L)												
Hypertension	Yes	Yes	Yes	Yes	Yes	No	Yes	Yes	No	No	Yes	No
Smoking	Yes	No	Yes	Yes	No	Yes	No	Yes	No	Yes	No	No
Diabetes	Yes	Yes	No	Yes	No	Yes	Yes	No	Yes	No	No	No
LVH	Yes	Yes	Yes	No	Yes	No	No	No	No	No	No	No
Age (yr)												
70	5·5	5·5	5·5	5·8	6·3	6·9	8·5	9·8				
68	5·5	5·5	5·5	5·8	6·4	7·0	8·6	9·9				
66	5·5	5·5	5·5	5·9	6·5	7·1	8·7	10·0				
64	5·5	5·5	5·5	6·1	6·6	7·2	8·9					
62	5·5	5·5	5·5	6·2	6·8	7·4	9·1					
60	5·5	5·5	5·5	6·4	7·0	7·7	9·4					
58	5·5	5·5	5·5	6·7	7·3	8·0	9·8					
56	5·5	5·5	5·5	7·0	7·7	8·4						
54	5·5	5·5	5·5	7·4	8·1	8·9						
52	5·5	5·5	5·9	7·9	8·7	9·4						
50	5·5	5·5	6·4	8·5	9·3							
48	5·5	6·0	6·9	9·3								
46	5·5	6·7	7·7									
44	5·5	7·5	8·6									
42	5·8	8·5	9·8									
40	6·7	9·9										
38	8·0											
36	9·7											
35												

Sheffield table for primary prevention of CHD

A patient whose value falls in the area with no entries has an estimated risk of coronary events of less than 3·0% per year

Notes on use of table

- Do **not** use for decisions on **secondary prevention:** patients with myocardial infarct, angina, peripheral vascular disease, or symptomatic carotid disease already have high CHD risk
- At this CHD risk (3% events per year) treatment with a statin (but not necessarily other drug classes) is justifiable
- The value of cholesterol reduction at <5·5 mmol/L or age >70 years is not established
- Use table **after** appropriate advice on smoking, diet, and control of systolic blood pressure to ≤160 mm Hg
- Use the **average** of two or more cholesterol concentrations
- Consider **individual** factors (eg, low high-density-lipoprotein cholesterol or bad family history), in final treatment decisions
- The table is valid for UK, Northern European, and North American populations—Southern European and Far Eastern populations have **lower** CHD risk in relation to the standard risk factors

Instructions

- Choose the table for men or women
- Identify the correct column for smoking, hypertension, diabetes, and left ventricular hypertrophy (LVH) by ECG
- Identify the row showing the age of the subject
- Read off the cholesterol concentration at the intersection of the appropriate column and row:

  If there is no entry, **cholesterol need not be measured**

  If there is an entry, **measure serum cholesterol**

  If the average cholesterol on repeated measurement is at or above the level shown, the CHD event risk is ≥3·0% per year—**consider treatment**

  The table can be used to **look forward** to possible need for measurement or treatment at an older age

Persons in the white part have a CHD risk of less than 3% per year, even if the blood cholesterol is very high. In this cohort, blood cholesterol testing does not make much sense. In Switzerland and Germany, the risk is only half of that in Britain and in the US. We can apply the Sheffield Table for women as well as for men.

Petr Skrabanek told us the following Persian story at the 1st Scientific Symposium of Einsiedeln 1993: *An old master is surprised by his young gardener who comes to ask him for his fastest horse) as he has to be away tonight. The old master asked him why he was so excited) has something happened? The gardener told him he saw Death while he was working in the garden) and Death threatened him. He realized he had to hide on a farm) otherwise Death would get him. The master gave him the horse and the gardener rode away to the farm. Later, the master was walking through the garden) and he also saw Death. He asked Death why did you threaten my gardener? And Death replied, "I was not threatening him. I just wondered what he was doing here as I was supposed to meet him tonight on the farm."*

This story nicely illustrates our modern problem with pathological findings. If every shady abnormal finding is seen as a threat that must be combatted, doctors and patients keep busy running away from Death – in a "folie à deux".

Therapy and therapeutic context

The discussion of therapy and therapeutic context leads us now directly to placebo in clinical trials. Alvan Feinstein put it forward at the 1st Scientific Symposia of Einsiedeln, that the role of the doctor is primarily to alleviate and comfort according to the old French aphorism: *Guèrir quuelque fois, Soulager souvent, Consoler toujours*. Feinstein was critical of modern medicine in that it looks down on the tasks of alleviation and consolation and limits itself to organ repair (the so-called apparatus error model). He emphasized the need of a nosology of placebo effects. The first time I had to deal with placebo in clinical trials was the acupuncture congress 1992 in Rome. I was faced with a few questions of how to design controlled trials for acupuncture. I found many studies using sham acupuncture, but this may be a wrong way to go. The doctor and his way of thinking may have a strong placebo effect. The instruments used (acupuncture needles) are perhaps merely vehicles of these effects. Because of technical difficulties, surgery does not generally use sham surgery as a control – there are only a few exceptions. The placebo control, in the end, is a method with questionable external validity in studies of acupuncture and many other techniques. The question of whether a given therapy is specific or non-specific has little other than theoretical value. The patient is interested how effective, sustainable, safe and costly a therapy is. *Bradford Hill* said in 1963: "If there is a treatment of accepted value, the question whether to use a placebo will hardly arise, for the doctor will wish to know whether a new treatment is more or less effective than the old, not that it is more effective than nothing" (quoted by *Kenneth Rothman* in an editorial with the title Placebo-Mania, BMJ 1996).

The questionable validity of placebo-controlled trials has barely been addressed by the new school of EBM, probably because a methodological confusion prevails. Many academics are hesitant to be identified with placebo effects, and they do not realize that the uncritical perpetuation of placebo controls is not in the interest of the patient. An elucidated understanding of placebo controls is not easy because conventional academic medicine is preoccupied with the concept that alternative medicine, such as homeopathy, chiropractic treatment and light therapy is quackery. Academic medicine ignores for the most part superstitious beliefs, although some inroads have been made. The instrument of the controlled trial by Archie Cochrane, no doubt, is the best standard we have to test therapies – entire therapeutic settings and pharmacological agents. The DBRCT is the best we have, but we must keep in mind that a placebo-controlled trial is a special design to test isolated pharmacological factors. Alvan Feinstein accurately demonstrated in his 1987 book *Clinimetrics* that there is a fallacious academic tendency to understand specificity as scientific evidence. Specificity, however, is often at the cost of sensitivity. Modern medical science is not always relevant for the practice of medicine. It is important to understand that clinical studies need to apply an intelligent compromise between the sensitivity and specificity of therapies. The literature describing pragmatic, practice-sensitive study designs is still scarce. Randomized trials (Simon 1995) or randomized trials with individualized therapies (Holle et Pritsch 1996) are common. The placebo-controlled trial is overly specific and not sensitive enough for practice relevance. The school of EBM does not seem to have internalized this.

Disease and disease context

It may be helpful to first address the question whether modern medicine has overcome and left behind exorcism. We have seen how much exorcism of threatening findings through cholesterol screening, for example, is flourishing. We tend to assume that exorcism, like treating patients based on blood cholesterol tests, can be useful. The problem is a fear-based instead of knowledge-based, no matter if we use old or modern techniques. The medical handling of cancer, similarly, seems to follow the priestly reflex to segregate the malign devil (the cancer) which is in fact also part of God's creation. Argument and dispute would be more helpful than segregation. Since the nineties of the last century there is ample evidence about the scarce effect of medical cancer cell removal as there is little effect of local cancer eradication on mortality (table 2).

Table 2. Breast cancer eradication and mortality.

Radical surgery	<->	minimal surgery	
no difference Local radiation	<->	no radiation	
no difference Minimal surgery	<->	no surgery	not known

All the traditional breast cancer treatments have severe adverse effects, but the ideas of treatment are rather mystical and there is a lack of good evidence that they do less harm than good. Feinstein has shown that the patient context, i.e. how is the patient able to cope with daily activities – is more important for the prognosis than histology and TNM stage. Some soft clinical interventions such as psychosocial support and palliative care could turn the disease from a malignant into a more benign course. Illness is always a product of disease and host resistance (figure 5). Conventional medicine focuses on supposedly objective diseases whereas complementary medicine and psychotherapy rather focuses on the host and education/ formation of the host. It appears that placebo has an effect on host formation. Whether host formation leads to a beneficial effect can be studied in pragmatic clinical trials just as much as it can and should be studied whether pathogenesis blockers – betablockers, antidiabetics, ACE inhibitors, serotonin antagonists etc. do more harm than good and in what context. In principle, the methodology for complex clinical trials exists today and it is evident that clinical research can and should study the great variety of interventions to find what is beneficial for the patient. It is of lesser importance whether it has a label of placebo or specific or somatic or psychic or functional therapy.

Figure 5. Disease context/illness as a product of disease, host and environment.

	50% Senkung		
Vorbehandlungs-Risiko *baseline risk*	————>	**Nachbehandlungs-Risiko** *post treatment risk*	**Number needed to treat**
100%	————>	50%	2
2%	————>	1%	100

Bildung = formation/education
Demographische Daten = demographics: ecological damage, climate, employment situation, religion, culture, education system
50% Senkung = 50% reduction

A pragmatic nosology

The modern clinical research methodology has already said farewell to the discussion about placebo and specific effects. There remains the difficult task to develop step by step a new nosology of the host and of disease contexts which allow prognostic information and the definition of which therapy is best indicated. We are quite confident that the work of a further development of a pluralistic EBM will be the future of medicine.

CHAPTER TWO

IS RENUNCIATION OF INTERVENTION ALWAYS NIHILISM? A RATIONAL MEDICAL PRACTICE BASED ON EVIDENCE

Preliminary remark: During my professional life, a number of essays and speeches occrued which all deal with the central aspect of modern medicine: the patient. As an author of clinical epidemiology and EBM, I increasingly realized that the main theme of EBM was the new look at the patient as the object of medicine. Supporting salutogenesis as much as fighting disease and pathological findings is the route medicine has to travel (again). The first time this issue became apparent to me was when I prepared an invited speech at The German Congress of Internal Medicine chaired by Johannes Koebberling. It was released in a book edited by Koebberling in Springer Publishing, Berlin 1998: „Zeitfragen der Medizin". Here is my English translation.

Speech by Johannes Schmidt delivered at the German Congress of Internal Medicine, Wiesbaden, April, 1997. First published in J. Koebberling. Zeitfragen der Medizin. Springer Berlin Heidelberg 1998
http://www.paracelsus-heute.ch/cms/literatur/PDF/Springer1997.pdf

The critical appraisal of scientific evidence in medicine is going through a striking transformation. Up until now, a pathophysiological improvement in the patient was considered evidence for effectiveness and patient benefit, but methodological progress has made it clear that we must also gather evidence of a reduction in morbidity and patient mortality and of improvement in the overall quality of life. The effect of the intervention must be significantly demonstrated, and expressed e.g. in the number-needed-to-treat. Such a rational and critical appraisal is often faced with the reproach of being *nihilistic.* To accept medical powerlessness and to engage in medical activism, meanwhile, could be the most important development of medicine in the coming decades. This is something, because we now have study results that show, for example, that breast cancer can lead to an improvement of the quality of life despite the physical ailment, as spiritual growth and consolidation of relationships occur.

If I consider the short time between my undergraduate medical education and today – just 15 years – a striking change in the appraisal of medical effectiveness and benefit has become apparent. In recent times, the catchword EBM is the term used for this change. The corresponding scientific methods of clinical epidemiology have been formulated for some time, but the rapid propagation of EBM seems to demonstrate that among many medical scientists, the notion has found acceptance that conventional university medicine has not been based on proper scientific evidence, but on credence and opinion.

Cognition and the corresponding nature of evidence

Of course, the medical community has attempted to base their doctrines on the available evidence long ago, but the methodological progress in clinical epidemiology has led to a change in the criteria of what can be considered as valid evidence. A positive change of laboratory or imaging findings was generally considered evidence of effectiveness. Now we request evidence of a beneficial change in patient parameters such as morbidity, mortality and quality of life. We further request results of controlled trials that show a difference in these parameters that is enough to result in a reasonably low number needed to treat (NNT). Physiological mechanisms of action are theorized, but they have a low rank in the current hierarchy of evidence.

I am aware that I speak to internists and specialists in internal medicine today. I can assume that the CAST trial is well known. This well designed trial has shown us how greatly we had been misled by pathophysiological reasoning that was based on insufficient studies suffering from selection bias. Uncontrolled cohort studies seemed to demonstrate that patients with ventricular arrhythmia had a far better prognosis if the arrhytmia was successfully suppressed by medicine. Arrhythmia which is easily supressable is not the same as arrhythmia that is not. No two patients are the same, and yet we hurtle headlong into categorization of patients in groups that can be treated the same. The cohort studies mistakenly compared different patients and not different treatments. CAST showed that the drugs could effectively supress arrhythmia and make the ECG look normal, but that mortality was 3-fold under the active treatment. CAST is perhaps the classic study to inform us of the surrogate fallacy, i.e. the observation that improving the ECG is not the same as an improvement for the patient.

What activities are possible in this time of methodological change? It is a very fascinating professioal challenge. You can choose to stay safe with the great majority of indifferent colleagues - which may in turn carry the risk of sitting suddenly on a historic steamboat instead of a modern jet. Instead, you could start to distinguish which evidence is solid and unbiased from lower level evidence which may be faulty, and to distinguish quantitatively important effects from effects which operate in 1 of 100 or only 1 in 1000 patients, and thus become irrelevant (see e.g. [3]).

Fallacies in the current management of cancer

I ask for your acceptance that I use oncology to illustrate the change of scientific reasoning. Cancer leaves no one aloof and creates emotions. It is often the reason for extensive diagnostic activities with little benefit. We must do all we can and apply every medical means, because otherwise we could be accused of nihilism. I want to provoke you and state that the medical management of cancer – I will use breast cancer as example – appears to follow a rather cultural reflex of devil exclusion rather than a careful consideration of biological evidence. If we have something that seems to be able to combat cancer, we have considered it as evidence. This proposition may be a bit black and white, but I use it for the purpose of elucidation.

It occurred to me that we should look back and consider the great success of modern developments in abolishing infectious diseases to a great extent. In table 1 I have compared breast cancer with tuberculosis. In the case of tuberculosis, we have learnt that the host condition matters. There are no aggressive and less aggressive tuberculosis bacteria, but differences in the host. The same we could assume for breast cancer cells. In fact, we know that there are healthy breast cancer cell carriers as autopsy studies reveal. The strength of the host may also matter in cancer and perhaps we can find more progress in this direction.

CHAPTER THREE

LOW LEVEL LASER THERAPY AND MYOFASCIAL PAIN

RICHARD EVAN STEELE

Abstract: An effective treatment modality leading to freedom from pain for whiplash syndrome, tension headache and post-concussion syndrome is presented. The background and theoretical basis of low-level laser therapy is presented. 5 cases representing patients treated with low level laser therapy are reported. The need for financing is discussed.

Keywords: inflammation, myofascial pain, whiplash syndrome, tension headache, post-concussion syndrome

Contributorship: there are not contributors

Funding: No outside funding

Competing interests: None

Acknowledgment: None

Introduction

There are at least 300,000 and possibly 500,000 to 600,000 Danes suffering from more or less chronic myofascial (myos is Greek for muscle and fascie is Latin for ligament) pain. This figure is gleaned from my experience as a municipal medical consultant with approximately 10000 cases over my table, where about half of these had myofascial pain syndromes as their presenting issue – whiplash syndrome, tension headache, post-concussion syndrome, lower back pain and many others. The number is derived by taking the percentage of the population locally and multiplying this by the total population. The most common and well-known examples of myofascial pain are whiplash syndrome, post-concussion syndrome, and tension headache. This is a very poorly researched area, and my observations are based on my own experience. Other less common myofascial pains include frozen shoulder, mouse arm, tennis and golf elbow, lower back pain, facet joint syndrome, groin pain, bursitis coxae, unspecific joint pain in general and unspecific muscle pain. I have been unable to find literature to document this. This also is based upon my own experience. All of these syndromes are characterized by a lack of specific treatments and so far, no generally applicable, effective solution has been described. Again here, there is no literature documenting this, but the issues are plain for anyone dealing with these patients. This article has 3 purposes. The first is to describe the importance of examining the condition of the muscles when facing patients with myofascial pain. The second is to describe low-level laser therapy (LLLT) as an effective therapeutic form for myofascial pain, and the third is to illustrate the effect of this treatment with some examples.

No one knows how many patients with tension headache have been diagnosed with migraine, but there is no doubt that this misdiagnosis exists. This is again one of those truths that everyone knows, but the no one has been able to document. This is one of the common elements of our methodology, that we are perfectly capable of documenting what we do right, but horribly incapable of documenting what we do wrong, is wasteful and/or deleterious for our patients. The main reason for this misdiagnosis is the lack of examination of the condition of the neck muscles, which is the cause of tension headaches. In my experience, none of the patients I have examined have ever had their neck muscles examined by any of up to 35 different doctors and other therapists. Examining the muscles of the neck, one can determine whether or not platysma, the scalenes and trapezius muscles have normal consistency or, as is the case with patients with tension headaches, have increased tension and often with myoses. It takes a little training to complete a sufficient examination, but everyone with reasonable fingertip sensibility, knowledge of anatomy and pathophysiology can easily learn to do a qualified exam of the tension status of the neck. Specifically, myoses on the medial scalene can cause visual disturbances that contribute to the misdiagnoses[1].

The examination technique requires palpation of the named muscles with a light hand, so that the muscle structure can be felt through the skin. It is decisive to examine the entire muscle. There is often a significant difference from side to side, which makes the discovery easier, as the difference is clearly felt. I find it most expeditious to do the exam on a gurney with a head holder so that the patient relaxes as much as possible during the exam.

Once such tensions have been established, there is a basis for referring to a clinic with experience in resolving the tensions. When the tension is resolved, the symptoms disappear. This is evidenced by my experience.

The past efforts have not been satisfactory. Although also not based in the literature, no treatment modality to date has been successful. The same applies to tension states that cause pain in other body parts than in the neck and in the head. It is clearly more difficult to detect tension in the deeper muscles, but a thorough history and prior examination with blood samples (exclusion of cancer, rheumatoid arthritis and vitamin D deficiency), ultrasound, X-ray, CT and/or MRI scan, which exclude more serious causes of pain, are usually negative in myofascial pain patients. When all studies show normal results, one can conclude that muscle tension and/or inflamed tendons and/or joints are the cause of the pain.

LLLT made its debut in Hungary in the early 1960s. A Hungarian surgeon Edre Mester (EM) has been credited with using it for the first time[2]. It was shortly after the ruby laser was put into use. During experiments with mice where he wanted to demonstrate the effect on induced skin tumors, which he could not detect. However, he noted a difference in the hair growth rate in the treated group compared with the untreated group[3]. Since then, attempts have been made to use LLLT over a number of conditions, of which myofascial pain is the area where the greatest effect is achieved[4]. There are numerous laser devices on the market, but the device that is best documented and with EU approval is LX2 from Thor Laser in the UK. LLLT has been the subject of study at the Harvard University School of Medicine, which has published an account of the mechanism of action[5]. It is a biphasic light source with a visible element of 720 nm and an invisible laser light of 613 nm. The visible light does not penetrate the skin, but the laser beam reaches 5-6 cm under the skin, depending on the tissue type[6]. There is no complete clarity on how it works, but there is no doubt that it acts as a powerful antioxidant locally. The role of antioxidants in reducing inflammation is well described[7]. It is less clear that myofascial pain is dependent on inflammatory processes, but what else should it be? How LLLT is anti-inflammatory is further described[8].

The muscles reveal varying degrees of affection by stress. It can be purely mental stress that affects the muscles and various physical stresses that become chronic pain syndromes. Head trauma, including concussion and whiplash, affects the neck muscles in varying degrees of severity as tension and/or myoses in the neck region. There is no obvious logical explanation for why post-concussion patients have the same tensions in the neck as whiplash patients, but that this is the case is clear to anyone working with both groups[9],[10].

A patient who could probably have been cured, but who could not afford the treatment, and where the municipality would not provide subsidies, is explained below. Most of us have met such patients, and the attitude is generally that one must learn to live with it.

A middle-aged man was hit some years ago by a car that did not yield as it should, while the man was riding on a scooter. The collision was so forceful that the patient was thrown over the car and landed first on his head, then on his left shoulder. The helmet he was wearing shattered. He was whisked to the emergency room, which did not find any broken bones or evidence of internal injuries, and he was sent home. In the weeks following the accident, the symptom complex that the patient was afflicted by developed. The symptoms are severe, constant back pain, left shoulder and upper arm pain, and fingers that sleep more or less constantly, which is most pronounced on the left side. In addition, he suffers from dizziness almost constantly, which is worst when he is tired, and frequent headaches. He needs rest often, but cannot find peace. He sleeps badly at night due to pain and tension, and must often rest during the day for that reason. From the objective examination: The body from the diaphragm and below is unaffected. The left arm can be moved slightly backwards, but not to the opposite hip. It cannot be pressed over the horizontal passively (due to pain) or actively. Good strength over the elbow, wrist and fingers. Right arm is normal. All the muscles in the neck are very sore, and with pronounced myoses in the playtysma, scalenes and trapezius, which are hard as wood on the left side and quite firm on the right side. Down the back, all muscles are very tense and hard from the top down to the sacroiliac joint, no soreness below this level.

This was a pronounced muscle-related problem with severe myoses, which had been attempted treated with physiotherapy and painkillers without effect. The condition is treatable with LLLT and massage. At least 30 treatment sessions would have been necessary, presumably taking 45 minutes per session although more treatments cannot be ruled out, depending on the result. The end-result would probably have been full recovery and return to workability, but at least a significant improvement would be achieved, and most likely a freedom from medication. The patient wanted to give the treatment a try, but since there was no financing available, the case did not continue.

Methods

Treatment with LLLT is delivered via a probe which is placed on the skin over the target muscle. It is not important that the skin is bare, but it does help to identify the underlying structures. The apparatus has two settings that are adjustable, that is the frequency of the flashes of the given light and the duration of the treatment. The frequency can be set from 2.5 Hz up to continuous over 12 increments, and the duration can be between five seconds and five minutes, also over 12 increments. Only two of the settings were used in this study, that is 2.5 Hz lasting 30 seconds, and continuous lasting two minutes. Treating a whiplash patient, which typically takes half an hour, typically includes a full treatment for all three scalene muscles, and varying portions of platysma and trapezius. These are treated with 2,5 Hz for 30 seconds per site. C3, C4, and C5 are given continuous light for 2 minutes per site. The probe heats up during use, but not to a dangerous level. It heats up to about 39°C before giving off as much heat as it creates. The tolerance of this heat varies extremely in patients. I switch between two identical probes so that one can cool off while the other is in use. A 40 mm probe delivers 1 W and penetrates 5 to 6 cm under the skin. A 65 mm probe delivers 1 W and penetrates approximately 1 cm under the skin. Experience dictates that treatment every other day is optimal. The duration of the treatment in terms of number of sessions varies extremely, from 10 to over 100 sessions until the patient is free from pain. Meanwhile, an average number is from 30 to 40. To date, no damage or side effects have been reported with LLLT. The only danger that has to be prevented is looking directly into the laser beam which can damage the retina.

Data Analysis

Simple collation

Results

There have been 178 patients in my clinic until now, and of these 25 with whiplash syndrome, 19 with post-concussion syndrome, and 23 with tension headache. All of these patients have become pain-free, none of them have relapsed. The rest of the patient population is a mix of various diagnoses, all of which have myofascial origins. There have been a number of scar tissue patients, and patients with eczema which have all improved significantly. None of the patients have continued with the same medicine that they took when they came to the clinic after ended treatment. This attests to the power of the treatment. Some patients have presented with pain syndromes that do not make any sense in a traditional medical model, but LLLT helped them nonetheless.

The following 5 examples will illustrate the effect of treatment with LLLT. These have been chosen to represent their case type. Any of the N=178 could have been chosen. The point is to illustrate the power of the treatment.

Patient No. 1 was a young man who had fallen off a horse 4 years earlier and had hit his head and neck and his back on the hard ground underneath. There were no immediate signs of major damage and no visible wounds. In the weeks following the fall, the boy developed a severe, constant headache, which was the subject of numerous studies. Among other things, a syringomyelia was detected at the L1 level, low pressure in the spinal canal and a moderate Scheuermann. None of these conditions could be linked to the headache. Various neurosurgical departments, pediatric wards and other specialists had found and accepted indication for treatment with Tradolan, Ibumetin and Paracetamol as well as Omeprazole to protect against the side effects of the Ibumetin. There was no focus on the neck muscles. On one out of approximately 100 pages of documentation in the case, there was one sentence describing the tense neck muscles by a physiotherapist. This passage did not have any consequence that one could glean from the documentation. When I met the patient, he had a very knotty neck, where especially the medial scalene was a chain of myoses, which was extremely sore. There were, as is usual for this type of patient, large myoses in trapezius both near the cranium and in the mid-clavicular level (MCL). After a series of treatments with LLLT and massage and the physical training I directed for the patient, he was completely free of the medicine and had a slight headache approximately once a week that did not require medication. His neck muscles were without myoses, but still a little tense. The treatment was completed 2 years ago, and the condition has remained pain free.

Patient no. 2 is a middle-aged man who 2 years before the exam in my clinic, was involved in a classic rear-end collision that hit the patient's car with such speed that neither of the cars could drive from the scene of the accident. The patient was wearing a seat belt and airbags were released. As usual for these cases, the primary examination at the hospital was without special findings. Approximately one year after the accident, the patient was awarded 8% disability and had been diagnosed with incipient dementia due to his reduced memory and concentration (common accompanying symptoms of whiplash syndrome). Again, no one in the process had examined the patient's neck muscles. When I met the patient, he had severe tension in the neck muscles and myoses in the medial and posterior scalenes as well as in the trapezius near his cranium and in the MCL. After a series of 32 treatments, he had become pain free, his neck muscles relaxed, and he had regained his memory and concentration. The treatment was completed 3 years ago and the condition has remained pain free.

Patient No. 3 was a young woman suffering from whiplash syndrome after two rear-end collisions. She had constant headaches, strained neck muscles and was depressed all the time. After a few treatments she felt much better, and her treatment could end after 9 sessions. The patient had no longer any pain and a relaxed neck. She had regained her energy and was happy again (an unusually short process). The treatment was completed 3 years ago and the condition has remained pain free.

Patient no. 4 was a middle-aged man who suffered a concussion of medium severity approximately 3 years previous to his appearance in the clinic. He had been examined by neurologists, neurosurgeons and his own GP and treated with various measures, including physiotherapy and strong painkillers. He suffered from severe, daily headaches, difficulty in concentration and memory and pain in the neck and back. His physical condition made him so depressed that he had seriously considered taking his own life. After approximately 10 treatments, his medication could be reduced. The headache and neck tension gradually disappeared. Life returned little by little, and after 40 sessions he could be discharged without medication and without pain. His memory and concentration had returned and he could get back to his working life. The treatment was completed 3 years ago and the condition has remained pain free.

Patient No. 5 was a middle-aged woman who slipped and fell on ice in the winter and hit the back of her head. She had a very bad time during the ensuing days. It went better for a short while, but after a few weeks, headaches and neck tension started. This increased over a couple of months and remained unchanged until she presented in the clinic about half a year after the accident. She had been at a pain center where they had put her on treatment with pain medication. In my clinic she was treated with LLLT and massage. It took about 7 sessions before she could feel any improvement, and after approximately 11 treatments, she could discontinue one of 2 painkillers. After approximately 18 treatments, she could stop using the other, and within a few weeks she was completely free from headaches. After 34 sessions, she had fully recovered and was able to go to work again. She was happy and cheerful again. The treatment was completed 2 years ago, and the condition has remained pain free.

All 178 patient records have the same level of documentation and follow-up. LLLT in the hands of an experienced clinician is an effective treatment for myofascial pain.

Discussion

A thorough knowledge of anatomy and pathophysiology is crucial. In practice, this means that one must be medically trained to achieve the best results. To date, there is no agreement on the effect of laser therapy in the literature, but in my experience. amazing results are obtained with this technique. In my clinic, there is thus a 100% success rate with whiplash, tension headache and post-concussion syndrome (N = 178 at the time of writing). Freedom from pain is the dependent variable. In spite of the documentation and the good experience, the treatment has not yet been taken on any payer's agenda in Denmark, so the treatment must be patient-financed, which excludes most people with chronic pain from the treatment. Most of the patients with myofascial pain have quite limited funds to pay with as they live either on sick pay, cash benefits or disability pension (evidenced by my extensive experience with these patient groups).

There are 3 main reasons why public clinics have not taken LLLT on the program. The first and most important is lack of knowledge of the therapy and its effect, which this article attempts to address. The second is the time spent with the individual treatment, typically half an hour, sometimes less, sometimes more. The third is the price of the equipment, which is around DKK 80,000.

LLLT is widespread in the UK, USA and Canada but not yet in the Scandinavian countries. Payment from public or insurance-based payers would allow many more to afford the treatment, thus bringing many back to productive lives that are now unable to work.

Notes

[1] Bexander CS. Hodges PW. Cervical rotator muscle activity with eye movement at different speeds is distorted in whiplash. Exp Brain Res 2012; 217(1): 67-77.
[2] Perrera, Judith. The 'healing laser' comes into the limelight: In: Riegel RJ, Godbold JC, eds Laser Therapy in Veterinary Medicine Hoboken NJ, USA Wiley Blackwell 1987:1-6.
[3] Hamblin MR. Shining light on the head: Photobiomodulation for brain disorders. BBA clin 2016; Dec. 6: 113–124.
[4] Chow R. Johnson, M. Lopes-Martins, R. Bjordal J. Efficacy of low-level laser therapy in the management of neck pain: a systematic review and meta-analysis of randomized placebo or active-treatment controlled trials. Lancet 2009; 374 (9705): 1897–1908.
[5] Ying-Ying, H; Chen, Aaron C-H; Carrol; James D; Hamblin, Michael R. Biphasic dose response in low level light therapy. Nonlinearity in Biology, Toxicology, and Medicine: 2009: 1-26.
[6] Ibid.
[7] Siti HN, Kamisah Y, Kamsiah J. The role of oxidative stress, antioxidants and vascular inflammation in cardiovascular disease (a review). Vascular pharmacology 2015; 71: 57-6.
[8] Bjordal JM, Lopes-Martins RAB, Joensen J, Iversen VV. The anti-inflammatory mechanism of low level laser therapy and its relevance for clinical use in physiotherapy, Physical Therapy Reviews: 2010; 15 (4): 286-293.
[9] Marshall CM, Vernon H, Leddy JJ, Baldwin BA. The role of the cervical spine in post-concussion syndrome. Phys Sportsmed 2015; 43(3):274-84.
[10] Evans RW. Persistent post-traumatic headache, post-concusion syndrome and whiplash injuries: the evidence for a non-traumatic basis with an historical review. Headache 2010; 50(4): 716-24.

CHAPTER FOUR

LOW LEVEL LASER THERAPY AND CHRONIC OBSTRUCTIVE PULMONARY DISEASE

RICHARD EVAN STEELE

Kliinikken Livet, Silkeborg, Denmark

To cite this article:

Richard Evan Steele. Low Level Laser Therapy and Chronic Obstructive Pulmonary Disease. Journal of Family Medicine and Health Care. Vol. 7, No. 4, 2021, pp. 105-107. doi: 10.11648/j.jfmhc.20210704.14

Abstract: A novel treatment modality for the treatment of COPD is presented. A patient story in which a patient was brought from a pulmonary capacity of 25% to a pulmonary capacity of 44% over a series of 13 treatments is presented. The patient in question had a concomitant improvement in quality of life that is hitherto unheard of in this patient category. This study was neither planned nor theorized. On the contrary, it came about due to a patient query that caught me by surprise. Where she was before the treatment unable to carry out many activities of daily living without assistance, she was after the treatment able to carry out nearly all her activities of daily living without assistance. A case for the dissemination of this effective treatment is made. Low level laser therapy definitely has its place in the treatment of any inflammatory process for which reason it is clearly relevant in the COPD sphere. Experience of the author in related fields is shortly presented as well as the political and financial aspects discussed. There is no doubt that low level laser therapy will enjoy much further dissemination in the years to come, and this article is a step in that direction.

Keywords: Chronic Obstructive Pulmonary Disease, Low Level Laser Therapy, Cost of Disease

Introduction

Every experienced clinician has met many patients with chronic obstructive pulmonary disease (COPD) in various clinical settings [1]. The prognosis is generally poor, going from bad to worse and ending in death [2]. Death in a COPD state is not a best-case scenario, because the patient with COPD is generally plagued by angst stemming from the fact that anyone lacking oxygen becomes afraid [3]. This well-known fact as a factor leads to a low dose Benzdiazopines being prescribed to ameliorate the angst condition [4]. The story described below is of a different nature, one that flies in the face of common knowledge and elucidates a methodology which can alleviate the burden for many COPD patients, while at the same time saving health care systems for billions in outlays that could otherwise be spared. Chronic obstructive pulmonary disease (COPD) is a widespread killer of, especially, older smokers of tobacco and/or previous heavy users. The economic burden of COPD in Denmark was estimated to be about EUR 1.13 billion in 2010 [5]. The authors of this article utilized good methodology to ascertain many various costs not readily visible for all, including loss of workdays, next of kin loss of workdays, transport to and from hospital etc. Obviously, any method to reduce this burden would be beneficial.

A 73-year-old woman had booked a time in my clinic due to back pain. The pain was diffuse lumbar pain with no neurological complications. On her first visit, the patient needed three pauses going from the ground floor to the level above, where the clinic is located, and had a slightly wheezing inhalation and a heavily wheezing exhalation which continued throughout the treatment which lasted an hour. The patient asked me if I thought that low level laser therapy (LLLT) could be beneficial for her COPD. The patient's pulmonary capacity had been measured some days before her visit to 25%. I told her that I did not know, but I knew that a significant part of the COPD condition is inflammatory [6], and I thought it worth a try.

Methods

The patient was treated sitting on the edge of the gurney, as she could not lie down flat, and the gurney does not have a raisable top half. The treatment consisted of adjacent pulses of low-level laser therapy consisting of five diodes emitting 200 mW each for a total of 1 W. All of both lung areas were treated thus which makes the treatment a time-consuming process. The diagnosis and the workup require medical knowledge and experience, but the actual application of the laser light could be administered by just about anyone given medical supervision. The laser element of the diode emits laser light with a wavelength of 613 nm as well as a visible red light of 720 nm. The unit runs on standard wall outlet power, and is compatible with both US and European voltages and frequencies. It has been established that the laser light emitted by Thor Photobiomodulation's LX2/2 laser apparatus penetrates tissue to at least 6 cm, although this was established in necrotic brain tissue [7]. It stands to reason that the penetration is greater the less dense the tissue is.

Results

LLLT has been shown to improve walking distance in a cohort of Egyptian COPD patients [8]. The Egyptians did not use spirometry, perhaps they did not have the apparatus. At any rate, the results were impressive. After 5 sessions, my patient was able to go up the stairs without pauses, and after 13 sessions, her pulmonary capacity was measured to 44%. Her quality of life had improved considerably, and she was able to carry out many functions she had prior to my treatment considered undoable. This included participating in garden activities, going to the toilet without assistance, enjoying eating instead of it being a chore and many other small things that those of us without serious COPD consider naturally doable. This level of improvement in quality of life has never before, to my knowledge, been published in the field of chronic obstructive pulmonary disease. The patient was quite obese and had large breasts, which of course reduces the amount of light reaching the inflamed tissue. It stands to reason that slimmer individuals would benefit more from the treatment. The patient chose to discontinue the treatment after 13 sessions, so I do not know whether further treatment would have bettered her condition even more. LLLT has been shown to be an effective anti-inflammatory treatment [9].

Discussion

A Hungarian surgeon called Edre Mester is generally credited as being the first to use light therapy in the clinical setting. Using a mouse model, he attempted to show an effect on induced skin tumors using a ruby laser, as his theory was that a significant proportion of the skin tumors was of an inflammatory nature. He did not detect any effect on the skin tumors, but noted a significant difference in the rate of hair growth which was higher in the treated group than it was in the nontreated group [10]. The universality of the treatment modality is hampered by various factors, the most important of which is that treating with LLLT always reduces the amount of medicine a patient need take which of course is deleterious to the financial concerns of pharmaceutical companies. These companies have huge resources and reach as well as political clout, and this would likely lead to backroom discussions between pharmaceutical company executives and politicians about keeping LLLT on the sidelines [11]. A second factor is a lack of knowledge among clinicians in the field. My own example will elucidate this. I ran a clinic treating chronic pain patients from 2005 to 2011. The clinic was mobile, i.e. we visited the patient instead of the patient being forced to come to our clinic. The clinic had a success rate measured in terms of getting the patient back to the workforce as the dependent variable of 63% [12]. This was in a group that had at least one and up to three different specialist opinions that had defined the patient as being beyond therapeutic reach. The clinic used myself as the attending physician, psychologists and an excellent group of relaxation therapists that utilize various methods among these cranio-sacral therapy. An example will illustrate the power of this intersectoral approach. Hassan had lived in Denmark for 10 years when he was referred to my clinic by the county authority. He had not learned Danish during that time, so the workup and treatment had to be translated by an interpreter. Curiously, it was quite difficult to get Hassan to explain what his physical problems were, because when asked what bothered him, he started by listing all of the various torture sessions he had been through. I explained to him that we cannot make this go away, but we could treat his symptoms and asked him what they were. He spoke of headaches and neck and back pains and pains in both shoulders. I asked my relaxation therapist to give him a treatment on the mobile gurney that we had along, and we removed ourselves from the room and had a talk with the wife and a son in the kitchen. After about 20 minutes, the relaxation therapist came out of the room and said that Hassan was sleeping. He appeared in the doorway a good hour later with a big smile on his face. The wife was flabbergasted, first because Hassan had a smile on his face, which was very rare, and that he slept for a full hour which he had not done since she had known him, sleeping only 10 minutes or so at a time. This of course was not the end of Hassan's problems, but it shows the power of addressing the symptoms rather than the story. This is typically what psychiatrists do in a procedure called incident debriefing [13] a procedure that retraumatizes the patient and has since been shown to do more harm than good (ibid).

The article (a novel and effective treatment modality for medically unexplained pain) led to me being recruited as the keynote speaker at the 2010 international conference on chronic pain in Jerusalem. This again led to me being recruited as the keynote speaker at the 2011 international conference on chronic pain in London. My lecture was followed by James

Carroll, the CEO of Thor Photobiomodulation who spoke of LLLT and its many uses in chronic pain. I was taken completely by surprise, as I had never heard about LLLT before then, and I am certain that if I had known about it while I had the clinic described above that my success rate would have been closer to 100% rather than 63%. I seriously doubt that if I had not been to this conference, that I would never have heard about LLLT. And when a specialist in the field has not heard of it, how can one expect others to gain such knowledge? At the recent PBM 2021, nearly all of the participants were LLLT practitioners, and the impact of such a conference is not very well disseminated in the broader clinical community. This in spite of the fact that we the practitioners generally do what we can to disseminate the knowledge that we have. Meanwhile, because of the issues named above we are fighting in uphill battle.

Conclusion

This study clearly shows that LLLT is an effective tool for ameliorating the symptoms of COPD, and casts a ball in the air waiting to be grabbed by the open-minded professional who is willing to entertain the prospect that this novel treatment modality has the potential to save thousands of patients from their low quality of life and give them back pulmonary capacity allowing them to do activities which they have been shut out from due to COPD. The treatment is time consuming and therefore difficult to sell. The treatment modality has the potential to save healthcare systems billions in direct and indirect costs, which should get payers to take notice.

References

1. Szalontai K, Gémes N, Furák J, et al. Chronic obstructive pulmonary disease: epidemiology, biomarkers, and paving the way to lung cancer. 2021 J Clin Med, 10 (13): published online without page numbers.
2. Ritchie AI, Wedzicha JA. Definition, causes, pathogenesis, and consequences of chronic obstructive pulmonary disease exacerbations. 2020 Clin Chest Med, 41 (3): pp. 421-438.
3. Tipton MJ, Harper A, Paton JFR, Costello JT. The human ventilatory response to stress: rate or depth? 2017 J Physiol. 595 (17), pp. 5729-5752.
4. Tselebis A, Pachi A, Ilias I, et al. Strategies to improve anxiety and depression in patients with COPD: a mental health perspective. Feb 9. 2016 Neuropsychiatric Treat., Neuropsychiatr Dis Treat: pp. 297-328.
5. Løkke a, Hiberg O, Tønesen P, Ibsen R, Kjellberg J, Jennnum P Direct

and indirect economic and health consequenses of COPD in Denmark: a national register-based study. 1998-2010. 2014 London British Medical Journal. 6 (4): pp. 237-246.
6. Chan SMH, Selemidis S, Bozinovski S, Vlahos R. Pathobiological mechanisms underlying metabolic syndrome (MetS) in chronic obstructive pulmonary disease (COPD): clinical significance and therapeutic strategies. 2019 Pharmacol Ther. Vol 198: pp. 160-188.
7. Clark E, Tedford I, Scott DeLapp I, Steven J, Anders J. Quantitative analysis of trnascranial and intraparanchymal light penetration in human cadaver brain tissue. 2015 Lasers in Surgery and Medicine. 47 (4): pp. 312-322.
8. Sayed MA, El-Sherif BM, Mohammed AR et al. Low-level laser therapy in chronic obstructive lung disease. 2018 Egyptian Journal of Bronchology. Vol. 12. pp. 317-322.
9. Steele RE Low level laser therapy and myofasical pain. 2020. New York, New York. Journal of pain mangement. 13 (1): pp. 56-62.
10. Perrera J The 'healing laser' comes into the limelight. In: Riegel RJ, Godbold JC, eds. 1987, Laser therapy in veterinary medicine, pp. 1-6.
11. Gaitonde R, Oxman AD, Okebukola PO, Rada G Interventions to reduce corruption in the health sector Cochrane, 2016, Vol 8 Cochrane Database Syst Rev, pp. 1-77.
12. Steele RE, Carpenter DO, de Leeuw E. A Novel and effetive treatment modality for medically unesplained pain. 2009 New York, New York. Journal of Pain Managemen. 1 (4): pp. 401- 412.
13. Foa EB, Gillihan SJ, Bryant RA Challenges and Successes in Dissemination of Evidence-Based Treatments for Posttraumatic Stress: Lessons Learned From Prolonged Exposure Therapy for PTSD. 2013, Psychol Sci Public Interest, 14 (2), pp. 65-111.

CHAPTER FIVE

TRADITIONAL CHINESE MEDICINE (TCM) AND CLASSICAL CHINESE MEDICINE (CCM)

Preliminary remark: Over the years I could increasingly rely on my practical work with Classical Chinese Medicine (CCM) which focusses on patient diagnosis and not on the disease.

TCM is not traditional, but was created during the 1900s. At the beginning of the 1900s, there were bad epidemics raging in China and the last emperor *Puyi* (1906-1967) forbid traditional folk medicine. He established new universities and recruited doctors of Western medicine to teach and practice modern Western medicine, which then became symptom oriented as in the West. Mao urged a revitalization of traditional folk medicine for economic reasons because Western medicine was too expensive for China. This was the start of TCM, now in the hands of Western-like universities and their symptom oriented thinking.

Classical Chinese Medicine, however, was patient- and recovery-oriented and focused on the patient diagnosis and his/her susceptibility to diseases and his/her weaknesses of self-healing and host resistance. This way of medical thinking and the corresponding Taoist masters, interestingly, existed at the very time of the European classical ancient time, in which physicians like *Hippocrates* (460-370 before Christ) and *Parmenides* (520-460 before Christ) laid the basis of Western medicine. Hippocrates emphasized the natural power of self-healing, which western doctors can only treat. It is nature that heals (medicus curat, natura sanat). This corresponds to the Taoist concept that man should only interfere in the natural course of disease with caution. *Parmenides* emphasized that fever is the sign of a natural healing process and therefore favorable for the patient. This corresponds to the "fire school" (*huo shen*) of the Chinese author *Zeng Qin-An* (1824-1911) who became aware that the old classical work of *Zang Zongjing* (150-250 after Christ), which contained a Taoist approach of being aware of the constant danger of losing the body. Yang gives cold a chance to invade the body. The world is cold and dark. Therefore, the body, Yang, needs to be protected and cared for. It is important to correctly diagnose "false heat" which is a result of cold damage and needs therapeutic warming and not cooling. *Master Hin Chung Got* (1946- 2021), who taught this practice to me, was a scholar of *Tang Buqi* (1917-2004) who edited the work of the above-mentioned *Zeng Qin-An.*

The great clinical significance of Yang, loss of Yang and maintenance of Yang is obvious in CCM. When Yang is too weak *Yin*, too, becomes endangered. Many fashionable medicines which are also administered by TCM doctors have a negative effect. While they adrenalize, they also exhaust Yang. False medicines of this kind are vitamins, algae, smoothies, energy drinks and transfusions of iron.

Beneficial sources of Yang are "grandmother foods" such as soups, well-cooked meat, especially beef, lamb and deer, shrimp and moderate red wine and grog, vegetables and spices such as onion, garlic, ginger, cloves, cinnamon, and "winter spices" – coriander, and herbs of dark and/or red color, rosemary, thyme, (brown) sugar, saffron, pepper and traditional broths with bones.

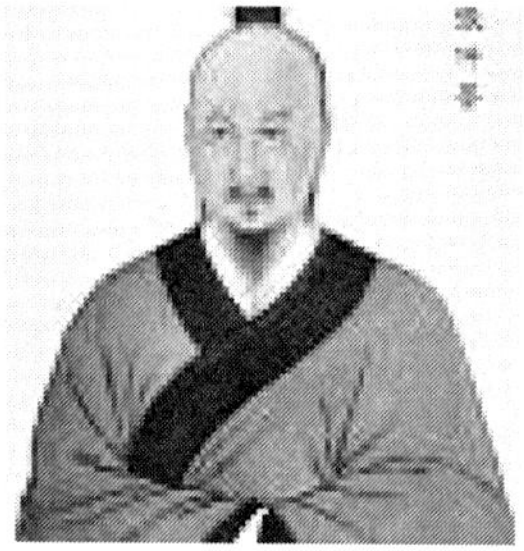

Zhang Zongjin

Dr. Johannes Schmidt, April 2020

Treat the patient, not his/her disease(s)

CHAPTER SIX

YANG-WEAKNESS AND DEFICIENT HOST RESISTANCE TO COLD – MAIN REASON FOR MOST CHRONIC DISEASES IN MODERN TIMES

Speech delivered at the congress of the Swiss Association of Acupuncture ASA, Solothurn 2014
http://www.paracelsus-heute.ch/cms/praxis/team/PDF/ASA_Vortrag_Skriptum.pdf

Why does one patient recover and another one not?

Wood

The topic of this congress is wood. In nature, wood is much more than a piece of wood. The classical Chinese view of nature is not a view of fragmentation. It remains important to see the forest behind the wood. Clinically, wood is the element of the fiercest symptoms, and such symptoms are often cured quickly. But is this all about Chinese medicine? The nature in classical Chinese medicine can be described as follows:

1. All is one – Tao. Clinical attention goes to perfection, more than to superficial suffering. Tao is composed of Yin and Yang. Without Yin there is no Yang. Without Yang there is no Yin. A visible deficiency of Yin in our patients is very often an (invisible) deficiency of Yang. For the human being, the world is cold and dark, and without a culture of Yang maintenance, man tends to lose his Yang.
2. Heaven – man – earth. In nature, man is between heaven and earth and is under their influence. Heavenly stems and earthly twigs determine the vagaries of nature and destiny. They can be stronger than our therapies. We should know them in order to distinguish

the subtle effect of the therapy, and

3. Rising – opening – sinking – closing: these four movements correspond to the 4 seasons. Rising is not just the contrary of sinking. If the center is missing the two movements can get in the way of each other. If a wheel has a functioning hub, however, the contrary movements can support each other.

Clinical Research, oriented towards patient benefit makes it clear that we will not only discuss the existence and nature of the placebo effect, but also the place of placebo in the context of clinical trials and clinical judgement. There continue to be debates whether placebo effects exist at all, but this can only draw attention to the fact that not every unexplainable improvement is a placebo effect. The natural course of the disease, maybe together with a regression to the mean, can lead to improvements, but in sum, this rather academic debate is of minor importance for our discussion. Often, placebo is called a non-specific effect. But it remains difficult to define what is specific and what is not (see chapters I and II). Placebo is rather well-defined as component of the placebo controlled double-blind trial, and its methodological place can be discussed. Of more interest is the fact that placebo, so far disdained as mere conceit and excluded from our clean clinical thinking, is being rehabilitated. Thus, a complete therapy of wood always includes metal and the center earth. The 4 phases include RISING (east = spring) – OPENING (south = summer) – SINKING (west = fall) – CLOSING (north = winter). For practical reasons and because of the great complexity of nature there was a need to add a 5th phase BIDING (center = late summer) The 5 elements, however, are not separate clinical boxes, but they produce and regulate each other in the originating cycle and the control cycle. They correspond to many natural phenomena such as seasons, color, cardinal direction, taste, but also the organs in which the invisible spirit of YANG is often clinically more important than the visible flesh of YIN. In the human body, eventually, we have 6 active layers: The 5 become 6 because we have two kinds of fire adding to the 4, the imperial fire and the ministerial fire. The 6 are: 1. cold water (TAI YANG), 2. aridity (YANG MING), 3. ministerial fire (SHAO YANG), 4 wetness (TAI YIN), 5. imperial fire or heavenly fire/light (SHAO YIN) and 6. wind (JUE YIN). I will now provide a short mention of the trigrams of the I GING mathematics. The barcodes of this classical Chinese science used in the I GING are more than the binary codes of modern computers. The relationship between these numbers and their origin matter in that ancestral lineage is thus explained. The thousands of phenomena in nature have all one origin, one root. This concept has its parallel in our Western science in that we understand that all matter is nothing but organized energy, although we do not begin to understand how gluons lead to the myriad forms that come from that one source, for not to speak of creativity, empathy and emotions. Analogue to a family there are codes for parents, grandparents, sisters, brothers, cousins and the many ancestors. They are related to each other and stem from one ancestor. Because of this complexity we always need a diagnosis of all organs, even if wood/liver produces the fiercest symptoms. A healthy WOOD can suffer if the mother WATER has a problem or if the center EARTH is too weak to hold the balance. In clinical practice we see basically 4 deficiencies on the horizontal or vertical axis, the liver-lung axis (balance) and the heart- kidney axis (connection/connectiveness) (see figure 1). The center/earth is always involved. EARTH should be strong enough to keep the balance and also be clear and strong enough to allow a good communication/connectiveness between the heart and kidney. Because a vertical axis problem also produces liver disorders, we need a clear diagnosis that makes it clear which organs need to be addressed by therapy. Wind can arise from heat (like in the desert) and heat can result from stagnation which often results from YANG deficiency, like a weak engine. For example, when a brain infarction produces the clinical symptoms of WIND, this is an irrelevant diagnosis. The root is Yang deficiency which fails to move the stagnation. The sole treatment of wood/wind would rather further debilitate the deficient Yang of the patient. If you support and strengthen Yang instead, the patient can recover. In cases in which wood/liver is a true basic weakness, you often need to treat the strategically important center/Earth Yang, not primarily the liver.

Let us look at a case: a 45-year-old patient came to see me 4 years ago. She suffered from nausea for over 2 years. She suffered from severe exhaustion. The medical record also mentioned some cachexia, amenorrhea and osteoporosis. She was depressed and hopeless, and she had a traumatic childhood. Since the age of 27, she got a disability pension because she was unable to work. The patient remembered digestive disorders since childhood, abdominal cramps and sometimes vomiting. At age 20 she contracted tonsillitis, and occasionally experienced a sense of a lump in the throat. And now she said, she was always freezing ever since, especially cold feet and hands. In July 2014, I diagnosed a very pale tongue and a rather weak pulse. The patient had back problems since age 32. Before the amenorrhea she had considerable premenstrual pain since age 27. She had been treated by a well-known TCM doctor in Zurich – with no improvement. Also, other TCM doctors prescribed complicated liver formulas and unfortunately vitamin infusions and very frequent acupuncture. In such cases one should do acupuncture not more than once every three weeks and use maximum 2-3 needles.

We can diagnose a severe Yang deficiency from birth. The parents were overstrained with the 4th child which we can call a Yang deficient cuckoo that was very vulnerable, with a weak center with weak self-confidence, weak lungs with oversensitivity, as well as a liverish sense of truculence and injustice. The difficult childhood is not a good diagnosis, but the congenital weaknesses are the true problem. We do not need a liver formula, but a firm Yang formula for the center – 90g fuzi, 90g dried ginger, 90g licorice (si ni tang). Soon after starting the herbal therapy, she had a crampy pain of the stomach though she had taken soy pudding which is contraindicated for a cold stomach. I took it as a sign that the frozen stomach began to wake up which was supported by the fact that the pain did not occur during the night. Afterwards, we had to deal with complaints of a dry mouth – still having nycturia two times nightly. When Yang returns, one starts to feel better. Dry mouth is the result of cold. The water in the body does not evaporate. The patient still had anxiety in the night, but sweating was already diminishing. After 3 weeks one could clearly see the marks and blood and damp stagnation on the tongue. Before, this was hidden in the ice appearance of the tongue. Nutrition which brings Yang to the body was important. Flatulence, at this stage, is an indicator of the growing digestive fire. A damp fire creates smoke until the fire gets strong enough to end smoking. Back pain increases temporarily, because also the back begins to wake up and later headache for the same reason. More important is the fact that appetite and eating improved steadily. As this demonstrates, the recurrence of pain while appetite improves is a good sign. Stool changed from loose to normal, almost dry. She became stronger and able to run again which helps improve sleep which also got better because the restless spirit found a warmer bed. From here, we must wait another 2 or 3 years for a consolidation and stable health.

The center

The middle/spleen is always the important target of treating Chinese liver disorders because a healthy liver-lung-balance needs a strong spleen in the center. The classical formulas such as danggui si ni tang, xiao chai hu tang, xiao yao san and chaihu su gan tang, indeed, all contain herbs that address and strengthen the center. The latter, however, I use rarely. It is a one-sided liver formula in modern times in which everybody has a weak center energy. CCM is strategic and primarily addresses the root (ben) and only if compatible also the pains (biao) if the herbs do not impair the root. An accurate look reveals that pains are often an indicator of the natural recovery process. It can be successful if we support the ben, the root. Nausea as we have seen in this case does not respond to herbs calming the liver, but with herbs to warm the entire body to help unfreeze the frozen stomach. The basic problem was a weak Yang as is often the case. Only heating herbs such as fuzi and gan jiang in rather high doses, tempered and harmonized by licorice, can solve the problem in this case. An ice clump can hardly be singed by the fire of toxic hot herbs. You need a high dose of fuzi, otherwise the ice will not melt. Licorice works like a pan between fire and water and allows the formation of steam and life. Where it is cold there is often a profusion of water. Foot edema, thus, does not respond well to diuretic herbs. You need to prescribe herbs to increase the kidney Yang which makes water evaporate and rise. Vapor invigorates and humifies everywhere. If there is water, the humid stays below and the result is dryness. Yang deficiency, thus, often leads to the false impression of dryness. But we know that the air is dry in winter, but humid in summer. A warm climate will help the earth to overcome aridity. "Don't drink a lot", my grandmother said, this will make you thirsty. My farmer grandmother in the countryside was still aware that drinking water stopped evaporation and resulted in a dry mouth. Prevent your patients from infusion such as vitamins or iron. We know the Chinese say that the blood must be cooked to become red. Infusions impair the fire of life and diminish the digestive fire which prevents deficiency. Indeed, properly controlled trials have shown that high dose antioxidant vitamins increase mortality and morbidity. Do not treat the liver and its windy affectation which stages the loudest and most agitated hype in the body. Treat Yang deficiency and the center/spleen – spleen Yang deficiency. Organs are just didactical entities. In fact, there is only one Yang.

Zeitgeist and old knowledge

The Yang school goes back to Zang Zhongjin 150-250 after Christ. But modern medicine tends to be panicky and inpatient. And the biao-oriented TCM likewise. This is the zeitgeist that facilitates the modern epidemic of chronic cold damage. The old books, however, enable a deeper look to the roots, to biao. Not only ancient Chinese medicine, but also our old books in the west draw attention to the primary importance of Yang. 500 years ago, Paracelsus, for example, reemphasis the significance of light as the basis for life saving.

"The right and true door to medicine is the light (of nature)"

Paracelsus did not say darkness and cold, but light which naturally is bonded to warmth and fire. After the time of Paracelsus there was a deep fracture in Western culture and development. Thanks to the undisrupted transmission of Asian medicine, however, we can still learn and understand this fire school from masters who have kept this school alive. In Europe, such biblical knowledge is now frowned upon. Medieval has become a synonym for terrible. Apparently, there was more continuity in Asia for reasons unknown to me. The clinical practice of the old Chinese bible *ShanHhan Lun* by *Zhang Zhongjing* is still known. I had the privilege to study it with my master *Hin Chung Got* (1946-2021). He had been a scholar of *Tang Buqi* (1917-2004) who had edited the writings about the fire school – huo shen – by *Zheng Qin-An* (1824-1911).

Cold damage, today, is rather the result of Yang deficiency than of exposure to extreme cold. A healthy body constantly gets rid of pathogen influences such as cold, mainly by producing fever and sweating. Yang deficiency can impair these reactions. Yang can be weak from birth (genetically) or by exhaustion or insufficient care.

False heat due to Yang deficiency

Cold damage causes inflammation such as multiple sclerosis (MS), polymyalgia, polyarthritis or hot flush. Furthermore, complementary medicine including TCM tends to treat such heat with cooling remedies because it is not understood that such problems are the result of cold damage. Inflammation and heat are mostly the result of cold. TCM takes it falsely as a Yin deficiency. I could relate a number of patient cases in which the warming treatment by Yang formulas caused a resolution of the inflammation and heat problems, sustainably because the true problem was addressed and improved with the result of a healthy resistance aging recurrence. We should see the principle that warming therapies resolve inflammation and cooling therapies increase (total) mortality.

Yang deficiency is a modern epidemic

The modern urban world is prone to confusion and gets too easily lost in false promises of improvement and progress, likewise in scholastic times of the late Middle Ages. Everything is a remedy or poison – it depends on the exact circumstances. Nothing is purely healthy or unhealthy. A balanced dose works different from an unbalanced dose. If we put a little grog into a fire, it burns well, but if we put a lot into it, it goes out. If we put a little fat into a fire, it also burns better, but a lot of fat would make it burn badly. The same with sugar. It produces a nice smell of caramel or extinguishes. Only in special burning devices we can burn rubbish, but not in the weak stomach fire of modern man. Vitamins, minerals, and other Yin substances can be digested and taken in the body if the digestive fire is strong enough. An overload of these substances is counterproductive unless the digestive fire is not well cared for by old-fashioned Yang nutrition. It is always of primary importance to strengthen and support the Yang. Many pains are then the result of a spontaneous clearing process in the body that maintains health and gets rid of cold pathogens. Fire can clean and clear. The purgatory fire, however, had been discredited in the late Middle Ages. Paracelsus, in his attempt to save this knowledge, said: "Every disease constitutes a purgatory fire. Therefore, no doctor can establish healing unless God foresees an end to it." If Yang holds, a patient becomes more mature and integrated after disease. The quantity of the single herbs is important for the effect of a classical formula. The blood must stay cool, just like lubricant in an engine, therefore we need Yin in the formula (e.g. bai shao) even if Yang is needed in a high dose. Pharmacological reasoning in the usual way is misleading: that 3g of Yang plus 1g of Yin results in 2g of Yang does not consider that in nature it is water and fire together that produces vapor.

Reasons for modern Yang deficiency

1. Top-heaviness – a lack of meditative activities weakens the spleen and digestive fire.
2. Alimentary fashions – cold and "wet food, iced stuff, drinking a lot, shakes, uncooked vegetarian food, soy, and so-called "supplementation" with vitamins, algae, ginseng etc.
3. Medical fashions creating early detection and screening illusions, reproductive medicine (fetuses with weak Yang), "freezing" of symptoms by cold or freezing medicines. Modern hyperactivity is rather the result than the cause of exhaustion.

Disease as a recovery process

We have seen some elements of improvements of basic strength and host resistance, and this may raise the fundamental question: Is the particular disease phenomenon the sign of a competent clearing and recovery process or rather the result of a failing resistance of the body, of incompetent Yang status? It is important to ask if it is a sign of strength or a sign of weakness and progressive decomposition. If you consistently attempt to understand the root of a disease and not only look at the superficial symptoms, growing practical experience will reveal the differences to you. You can hardly learn it from books. I have prepared a list of symptoms and clinical phenomena and their differentiation at the end. This table is tentative and preliminary, please do not quote from it. I want to point out the example of metastases because I have seen that even metastases can be a recovery process. A breast cancer patient of mine developed high fever after having had a pathological bone fracture because of bone metastases. She felt so ill that she decided to go to hospital to die. Radiotherapy helped to ease the pain. She declined chemotherapy which I think was a good decision. Eventually, the tumor fever established a process producing some painful blisters on the skin, a sign that cold left the body, making small frost boils. Herpes-like red blisters are taught to be a healing sign in ancient Chinese medicine. Pulse palpation and tongue appearance remained good. My master God had always taught me that Heaven determines the course of a disease and that we should remain patient. The remaining spirits will decide the outcome. I did not tell the patient that she would not die, I said that I am not God and cannot do much, but I said that her tongue and pulse looked good. After 3 days, the patient decided that she wanted to live. She got up and left the hospital to go home. She then had a good appetite which brought her back to power and strength. She had not lost her life, but only her fears – she got a firmer voice due to the new heartiness. After 6 months, she was still in good health and all signs of tumor and metastases (blood and x-ray) had disappeared. We observe often that pathological problems spread to both sides of the body when recovery becomes effective. It may be, therefore, that the spread of metastases is a tactic of the body to disperse tumor mass so as better to overcome the tumor. It may also be that metastatic cores are already there at the time of birth. Metastases are more often primary rather than secondary, as we know today.

Table 1. Note: these observations are from Dr. Johannes G. Schmidt and are preliminary. They should therefore not be quoted.

Symptom	Strong cleansing	Weak overloaded chocking
Flatulence	Comparable to a fanned fire in wetness that smokes until the flames get through – the flatulence is well tolerated.	Comparable to a suffocating fire, that starts to smoke – the flatulence is detrimental.
Cold feet	Under increasing inner fire (Yang), it gives way to cold feet and legs, possibly. Increase in calf cramps, nocturia decreases.	The lack of inner fire (Yang) leaves increasing cold in the body with the consequence of cold feet, possibly also with leg cramps, nocturia increases.
Warm feet	Heat dissipates and cold comes back.	Almost always a sign of cold on the way, the heat disappears.
Constipation, difficult defecation	Increasing warmth (Yang) in the abdomen leads to stiffer stool that is strenuous to empty because the warming/strengthening of peristalsis lags behind – with a good appetite.	Increasing constipation by increasing Yang weakness - more uncomfortable cold accumulation with loss of appetite.
Diarrhea/runny stool	Cold escapes from the middle, mostly only 1-3 x diarrhea per day – abdomen relatively pleasant, appetite good, usually only briefly disturbed. Cold overruns the middle and the evil.	Cold overruns the middle with nausea, abdominal cramps, and pains.
Joint pains	The warming body pushes cold/wet from	Joints assimilate cold throughout the body. It

	the joints, which hurts and gives severe pain. When the "ice breaks" dissipates- good appetite and sleep affected lightly	takes over and increases heat and inflammation causes pain - appetite and sleep are usually affected
Finger pains	Evasion of cold in the neck and/or shoulder temporarily causes pain in the fingers/hands without deformation.	Lengthy cold in the neck and/or shoulder leads to increasing pain in hands/fingers – with deformation and headaches.
Headache/migraine	Migraines are a symptom of exhaustion. With a good course the stronger body feels the load limits and can cope better.	With increasing weakness, migraines increase as an expression of the body not being able to cope.
Fatigue	A warm body gets pleasantly tired, the tiredness becomes clearer – and sleep improves.	A cold body does not allow better sleep, it becomes powerless and tired.
Metastases	Inflammation mobilizes congenital disturbances (primal cold) – and can via a tumor fever (with painful skin blister formations of the fever blister type) escape from the body	Failed attempt at self-healing overwhelms a weak resistance and leads to death.
The influenza and influenza induced long term effects	Eliminates invading cold via fever and sweating and restores health again – also triggers elimination from old cold.	When the defenses are too weak/blocked no real fever and sweating are induced, and the infection has few symptoms. It runs and remains as a burden in the body – or can cause

		death when resistance is too weak.
Night paleness	An alert mind may be temporarily stressed by the accepting challenges.	It is a sign of stress, usually an imbalance in the wood/metal condition.
Thirst	Genuine thirst with Yang strength depends on physical performance and sweat.	False thirst manifests from a dry mouth from internal cold, in which the water is not evaporated but humidifies.
The influenza and influenza induced long term effects	Eliminates invading cold via fever and sweating and restores health again – also triggers elimination from old cold.	When the defenses are too weak/blocked no real fever and sweating are induced, and the infection has few symptoms. It runs and remains as a burden in the body – or can cause death when resistance is too weak.
Night paleness	An alert mind may be temporarily stressed by the accepting challenges.	It is a sign of stress, usually an imbalance in the wood/metal condition.
Thirst	Genuine thirst with Yang strength depends on physical performance and sweat.	False thirst manifests from a dry mouth from internal cold, in which the water is not evaporated but humidifies.
Heat	Yang build-up can occasionally create false heat.	Increasing cold turns into heat, motivates feet out of bed, then covering up, nightly thirst, etc.
Urination issues	Disturbing urge to urinate when cold escapes via the bladder – without an increase in nocturia, burning	Chronic dysuria with urination problems and increasing incontinence.

	with micturition, frequent urination, nocturia – is basically also a clearing up process in the case of an acute cold or influenza.	
Cramps or sharp pain	Blood stagnation, scar pain when penetrating through a new location, e.g. at muscle insertions, chest, abdomen – can be very violent, usually only seconds or minutes or a few days to 3 weeks without any significant appetite or sleep disturbance.	Location stagnation increasing and the general condition impaired or sometimes with fatal complications, e.g. a heart attack.
Dizziness	With increasing strength of the middle (spleen energy) dizzy spells may occur in the sense of being shaken up. One may pause and find oneself – appetite not usually affected.	Increasing weakness associated with dizziness entails nausea and loss of appetite.
Hot flushes	The flush overrides liver control, and one can relax so as not to give a homemade gift to oneself, as the solution and this strengthens the center.	Middle weakness can equalize between liver rising and unregulated pulmonary sinking. This leads to increasing mid-fatigue in endless waves.
Depression	Unpleasant and painful sensation that something is wrong. Notions and beliefs do not correspond to reality and are not fulfilled – brooding	Unpleasant and painful sensation, those with increasing Yang depletion (darkness) do not fathom what is missing and the condition can become

	leads to "stretch out the feeler" and in Yang construction (light) finally to recognize another friendly reality (may take months or sometimes even years).	chronic (antidepressants suppress the Yang and make redemption difficult, at best).

I will now use an example of metastases to further elucidate the hypothesis that even these can represent a healing process. I experienced this recently with a breast cancer patient with extensive bone metastases, which included a pathological femoral neck fracture which led to pain relief and radiotherapy and a type of chemotherapy she had always refused, which probably was decisive. A few weeks later, she developed a persistent high fever and got deathly ill, and after three weeks of this finally went to the hospital to die. The fever seemed, however, to be a healing fever. The body was sick because it resisted and made painful blisters on the skin which caused the skin to come off under the blisters. Her pulse, tongue and appetite remained good. I didn't tell the patient they were not going to die, because my teacher Hin Chung Got had always pointed out that Heaven dictates that we must wait. Decision becomes the spirit of life. Dying is always the beginning of a birth, we know that well from the Chinese Seasons Analogy. Erich Fromm puts it such: "The goal of life is to be born whole, and its tragedy is that most of us die before we are quite born." I took it to mean that I should let time work instead of interfering as a doctor. I just told the patient that her pulse and tongue stayed well, and it was clear to me how it would turn out. Three days after her wish to die, she changed her mind and decided to live – she opened the coffin lid again, so to speak. She got up, left the hospital, and became extremely hungry. Her fears died. Her voice became firmer as an expression of what had been won – courage – the concurrent intact heart-kidney coordination, for which death is no longer a threat. Fear consumes strength. Overcoming fear makes resistance and recovery force available.

She has been vital and in good health for six months now. Her condition with metastases – or what is left of them – hardly hurt anymore. We see that blockages and especially cold blockages in the extremities distribute to both sides during recovery. Perhaps metastases are a tactic used by the body to redistribute the disorder to make it easier to get rid of. It can also be that the cold nests are genetically distributed throughout the body – we have learned that primary metastases are more the rule than the exception.

Consequences for clinical research

In closing, we challenge you to embrace a new paradigm for clinical research: The individual variation in the ability to recover applies to the patient accurately and enables us to treat the host and not his symptoms or diseases. If we view the lack of good digestion, sleep, and vital warmth – Yang deficiency – as the central characteristic in patients with MS instead of understanding the disorder only as a peripheral syndrome, we will require a different research approach. This would lead to the conclusion that many MS patients can become well. The conventional research approach is almost always about containing the symptoms of illness. EBM guides us to the question of health gain and relevant clinical criteria for success in a broad sense. Clinical practice and clinical research must therefore constantly ask the question: how is the whole host faring under the intervention (not only the disease and its main symptoms such as the neurological disorders in MS)?

Clinical knowledge of Chinese medicine can help us develop a more sensitive nosology and more effective therapies for the patient and not just against symptoms and diseases.

CHAPTER SEVEN

SUSTAINABLE MEDICINE OR SUSTAINABLE HEALTH?

First published in Swiss Medical Bulletin (Schweiz.Ärztezeitung) 2014
http://www.paracelsus-heute.ch/cms/literatur/PDF/SAeZ2014__NachhaltigeGesundheit.pdf

Why and when does a patient remain diseased and not recover? In fact, this is a central issue of evidence-based medicine EBM. The scientific question of clinical success is about the patient's abilities and wellbeing rather than about the pathological conditions and findings.

The entire world is diseased because we only speak about diseases and as a consequence have forgotten about health.
Foundation Paracelsus Today

In a paper on sustainable medicine, issued in 2012, the Swiss Academy of Medical Sciences SAMW raised the truly important question: Instead of addressing sustainable medicine, should one rather address sustainable health? "No", the authors said, because medicine is limited to medicinal issues and health is a political and social matter. This inspirational text lists the factors that may lead to life-long, non-sustainable maximal medicine. However, without addressing health as the issue, the reason behind these factors gets lost, as they are bound to the concepts of war on disease and the abolition of pathogenesis. The error of the current medical reasoning is that health is produced by this war and the abolition of pathogenesis.

What about health and salutogenesis?

We do not need a clear definition of health in order to address sustainable health. In our medical practice, we know what is meant by the following questions: Is health impaired? Did the health status change? Can we improve it? What about sustainability? Health has always been an issue in medicine, and EBM has explicitly brought it to the scientific table with questions regarding clinical endpoints which are relevant for the patient, and which allow a valid answer to the question of patient benefit. Meanwhile, it is true that medical practice continues to limit itself to diseases and pathogenesis, because it is believed that this has been the source of medical progress. It is overlooked that many diseases are attacked by our immune system and mental powers to a lesser or greater degree and are attenuated by a spontaneous recovery process. Furthermore, pathological findings and test results can give a false positive result due to natural variation. There is no definite boundary between diseased and healthy, and even true positive disease-findings can be compatible with good health, so that a growing number of healthy people and people in successful self-recovery are labelled as diseased by medical practice. This gives rise to many unwanted consequences of overdiagnosis and overtreatment, which is a matter of growing concern (Welch, Schwartz, Woloshin 2012). Politicians and economists have reacted by demanding limitations to such unhealthy medical practice. Such unhealthy medical practices are ineffective and counterproductive because common medical reasoning needs to be corrected. Modern medicine has gone through a strong tendency to sub-specialize where everyone sees their mission as an attempt to make war on diseases and pathologies with all means – with "maximal medicine" as the SAMW calls it.

Cosmetic improvement of diseases does not always confer a health benefit

The current medical reasoning also follows the error that the abolition of diseases automatically will improve health. Take the glitazones as an example. When they were introduced by the pharmaceutical industry, doctors got a powerful tool to improve blood glucose in diabetics and to achieve very good glucose values, as measured by HbA1c values. But the studies had not examined how the drug affects the entire patient. Years later, important endpoints were included to show that this successful drug increased mortality 4-fold. The medical community used the promising drug extensively without demanding a true scientific study with relevant endpoints. They should have known about this issue because in 1989 the CAST study had shown that a very successful treatment of irregular heartbeat by a new drug had harmed the patients by increasing total mortality 2-3-fold. The all-important question is whether a therapy has a beneficial effect on total morbidity and total mortality. Breast cancer screening, for example, can reduce breast cancer mortality to some extent, but total mortality remains unchanged (Schmidt 1990). We also know that the popular multiphasic check-up has no proven effect on total mortality and morbidity, the only difference is an increase in hospital admissions due to overdiagnosis (Cochrane Library 2012). The disease-based reasoning in medicine has a long tradition. Only a few decades ago, dying was considered a natural thing and took place in the community and family. Patients were not severely diseased except in hospitals. When the modern diagnostic technology became available, despite the new insights into the pitfalls of medical decision making (Sox et al. 1988), doctors started to use diagnostic technology in low diseased groups such as patients in their home or for screening healthy people without giving attention to the rules of low pretest likelihood and the consequences of false positive results. The euphoria over the technological improvements did not allow us to realize that most improvements in clinical disease courses were the result of natural, spontaneous recovery. It is common to refer to good courses without taking it into account that this was a selection of the good cases. This constituted a selection bias and not medical progress. Tuberculosis is perhaps the most pertinent example to show that the medical community occasionally understands the important role of the host. It became clear that it was not variations in tuberculum bacteria virulence that determined the clinical outcome, but variations in host conditions. The drastic decrease of tuberculosis was the result of clean water, sufficient nutrition and warm housing which became possible due to advances in agriculture and housing. This erroneous thinking, however, is deeply entrenched in the medical community. The most recent case of such an error is the COVID vaccine. There was good proof that the new vaccinations are effective in producing antibodies, but it was not examined whether that has an effect on the patients' resistance and susceptibility to infection. Many governments in Europe were foolish enough to promise absolute protection with the vaccination and declare it compulsory for everyone, without considering susceptibility to infection. The entire medical community, with the exception of the German Cochrane working group who drew attention to the radical lack of it, ignored this lack of evidence (Prof. I. Mühlhauser). It was brushed aside. The COVID epidemic was a dramatic example of the scientific ignorance of maximal medicine and of uncritical medical practice as well as an example of the ignorance among the European medical and political communities of epidemiology and the rules that govern EBM.

Treat the patient, not the disease

CHAPTER EIGHT

EVIDENCE OF EFFECTIVE DISEASE PREVENTION IS NOT YET PROOF OF HEALTH GAIN – THE PATIENT AS THE HOST OF HIS/HER DISEASE(S)

Speech delivered at the Medical Society of Basel ("Medges") 22/01/2015
http://www.paracelsus-heute.ch/cms/praxis/team/PDF/MedGes_Vortrag.pdf

Modern conventional medicine mainly follows a classification of diseases – everything is about diseases and abatement of diseases. The crucial determinants of disease courses, however, is the disease and the host or more completely the disease, the host and the environment (figure 1).

Figure 1

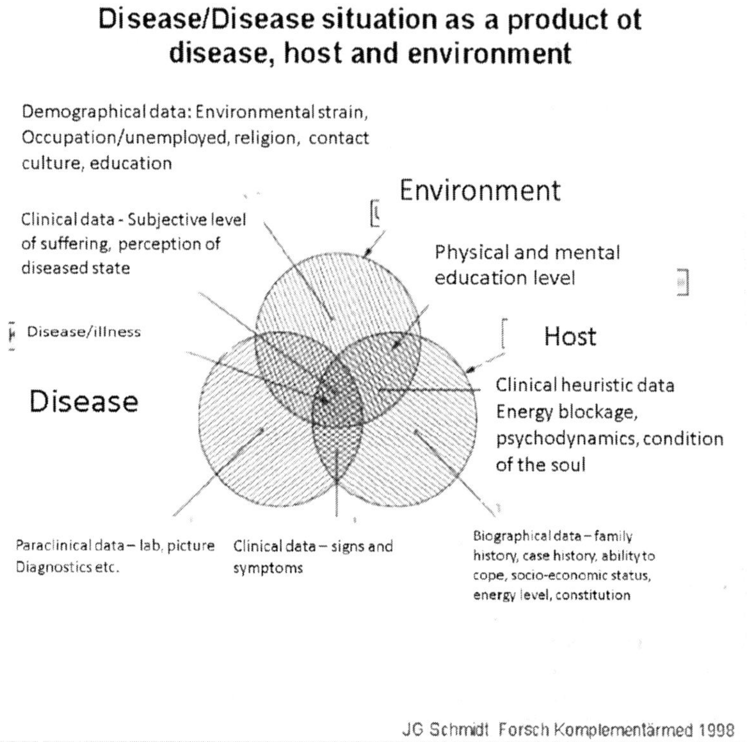

Ill health, therefore, is not just the result of a disease, but of the disease and the host condition. Consequently, one is not necessarily ill with a disease, and without disease one is not necessarily healthy. Good and sound medicine goes for diagnoses and treatments only if it is for the true benefit of the patient, avoiding overdiagnosis and overtreatment. We have to ask if diagnoses represent the true patient problem or if they rather mislead us to unnecessary or irrelevant medical measures. This is mainly the case in preventive medicine, but also in the case of the many interventions in terms of secondary and tertiary prevention. Indeed, we speak about quaternary prevention today, about the need of the prevention of iatrogenic harm. General medicine, indeed, may be considered as the specialty of the entire patient which consequently needs to focus on the interaction between pathogenic and salutogenic processes. The usual diagnoses according to the ICD classification, therefore, are an insufficient basis for medical activities.

We need a diagnosis of the patient situation (figure 2) which includes host resistance and individual recovery potential as much as the pathological findings.

Figure 2

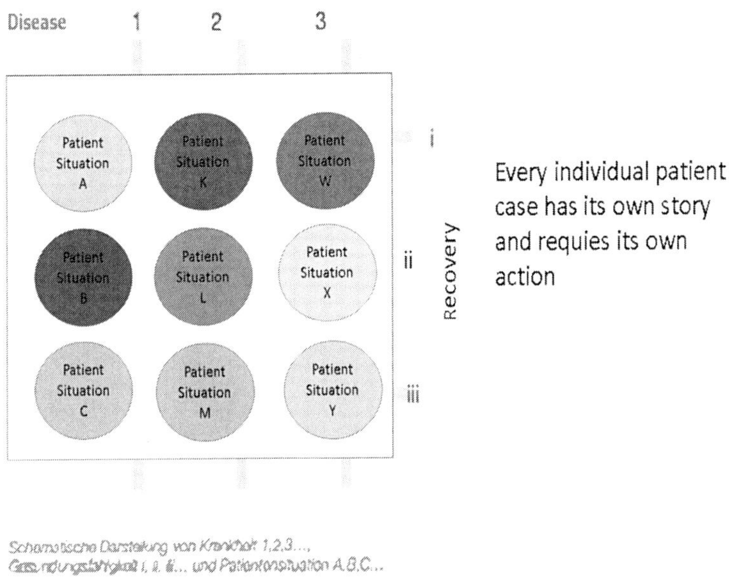

If we consider the traditional logic of medicine addressing the host as well as the disease, we begin to understand what we have forgotten in the last 100 years or so. Host resistance as well as the disease pathology determine the clinical course. 100 years ago, we were still aware of the role of the host. In fact, improvements in the host situation, i.e. proper food availability and warm housing, have made tuberculosis disappear. In the case of tuberculosis we have abandoned well-meant, but useless preventive measures because we understood the lack of benefit. If the concept of disease and host would not have been forgotten, there would not have been established so many preventive follies which now need to be abolished again with considerable difficulties. Meanwhile, we speak about quaternary prevention, which is the prevention of iatrogenic harm through overdiagnosis and overtreatment. We need to create prevention of preventive medicine. Let us look at the cholesterol story. Colleagues from preventive medicine, together with lipidologists have created a new disease – hypercholesterolaemia – that allegedly would need screening and treatment. If we look at the legendary

Framingham study, however, we can ascertain that also low cholesterol levels can be associated with later infarcts and that low cholesterol levels do not necessarily protect from later infarcts (figure 3).

Figure 3

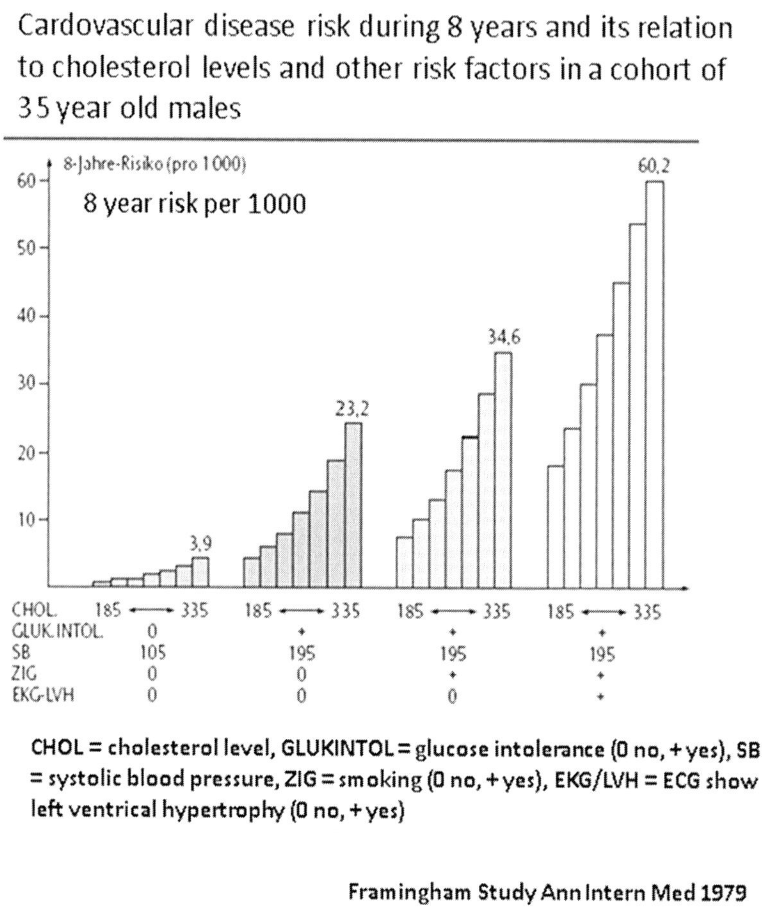

Men of age 35 can be grouped in those with no pre-existing problems (on the left) and those with pre-existing problems (on the right). In the host on the left the cholesterol level makes little difference in risk whereas in the host on the right, the cholesterol level makes a visible difference. Thus, a healthy host has no problem with an elevated cholesterol level. A previous infarct or the cumulation of many risk factors in the pre-diseased host show a problem of the host organism with elevated cholesterol levels.

Figure 4

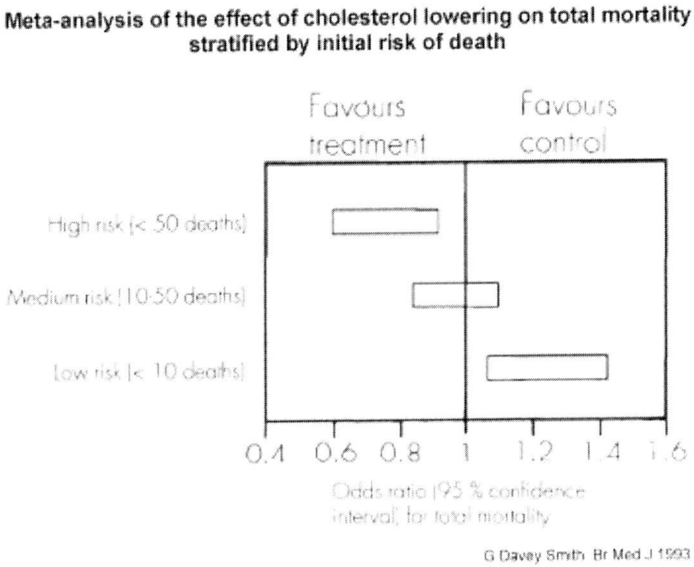

Figure 4 depicts the study of Davey Smith 1993 and shows not unexpectedly that cholesterol lowering treatment is harmful in healthy hosts (lower bar), and only beneficial in pre-diseased hosts (upper bar). Thus, primary prevention has increased mortality. That is far more the case than in secondary prevention. Before the statins, doctors have killed a considerable number of healthy people through so-called primary prevention – because we combat diseases without thinking about the great variation of host recovery potential. Primary prevention was established despite the fact that it had been proven harmful. The meta-analyses of primary prevention with statins show a difference of 1 death in 1,000 treatment years (table 1).

Table 1

Cholesterol lowering (Statins) and mortality, primary prevention

Ray K et al. Arch Intern Med 2010 — 3.7 years Follow-Up

	Participants	Total Deaths	per 1'000	per 1000 years	
Statin	32623	1346	41	11	No significant difference
Placebo	32606	1447	44	12	

Cochrane Collaboration 2013 — ca. 5 Jahre Follow-Up

	Participants	Total Deaths	per 1000	per 1000 years	
Statin	24408	1077	44	9	No significant difference
Placebo	23652	1223	52	10	

From a practical point of view, we must realize that one can also die with a statin (in 9 instead of 10 cases in 1000 treatment years); and one can survive without a statin (in 90 instead of 91 cases in 1000 treatment years). The Swiss Medical Board, consequently, recommended in 2014 that primary prevention should no longer be offered and pursued. Conventional medical reasoning dictates that treating pre-diseased hosts should be done more often, even if the cholesterol level is normal. We should abandon cholesterol screening. It is a strange error of modern medicine to misunderstand elevated cholesterol levels as a threatening disease needing detection and treatment with the result of worrying and ultimately killing a lot of people. There is no such thing as pathological and healthy cholesterol levels. Keep in mind the interaction between diseases and the host. A healthy host with a healthy regeneration has no problem with high cholesterol. A host with a deficient regeneration, however, has a problem even with a normal cholesterol. What now, is the natural course of breast cancer? Table 2 shows the lack of difference between women surviving breast cancer with and without breast cancer screening.

Table 2

Number of cases with or without mammography screening

In women aged 50-60 over a ten year period

	With mammography	Without mammography	Difference
Total mortality	76	76	0
Breast cancer deaths	3-4	4	0-1 (increase)
Diagnosed breast cancer	24	19	5 (decrease)
Total survival	924	924	0
No death from breast cancer	996-997	996	0-1
No breast cancer diagnosis	976	981	5
Number of mammographies	5000		
Suspected cancer	200-500		

There is a very small reduction of breast cancer deaths, but no reduction of total deaths. For the host, the death rate remains the same. At the same time there is an increase of diagnosed breast cancers of 5 in 10,000 screening years. And several hundred positive mammograms. Table 3 shows the results of an autopsy study in 1984. As you can see the great majority of breast cancers (70%) remain undetected during lifetime. Clinically appearing breast cancers do not cause death in 50% of the known cases. This is a constant figure over many decades. Survival in this group is 70% today, mainly because of overdiagnosis of healthy women through mammography screening and because of improvements in hormone therapy.

Table 3

How deadly is breast cancer? 83 unselected cases documented by Nielsen et al. Cancer 1984

Malignant cells at autopsy (in situ and invasive)	Diseased during life	Cause of death breast cancer	
21	6	3	
25%	7%	4%	All women
	29%	14%	All breast carcinomas

The question is: is it breast cancer that determines later death or are there other factors determining the outcome? Is it prudent to think of aggressive and less aggressive types of cancer cells? I think not. The idea that the host makes the difference is more plausible to me. In 1987, I could present the following table at the German Congress of Internal Medicine, "Internistenkongress" (table 4).

Table 4

Disease	Agent	Host	Mortality	Therapy
Breast cancer until now	Malignant cells (greatly variable malignancy)	Susceptibility unimportant	Unchanged for decades	?
Tuberculosis	Mycobacteria tuberculosis (virulence unchanged for centuries)	Susceptibility depends on host resistance	Decreases as housing and nutrition improve	Housing and nutritional improvements
The future of breast cancer	Malignant cells (greatly variable malignancy)	Susceptibility depends on our ability to increase the frequency of the healthy bearer	Improvement by improving spiritual health	Sanitizing the inner house, spiritual nutrition (salutogenesis)

JG Schmidt in Köbberling Zeitfragen der Medizin, Springer 1997

In terms of a practical breakdown of the methodology for improving spiritual enablement, table 5 can be helpful.

Table 5

Clinical anamnestic signs of improvement in basic strength
Signs of improvement - this can take years

Digestion	• Go for a balanced appetite without cravings • Discomfort and cramps due to the stomach awakening • More frequent bowel movements with a possible phase of sluggishness • Better tracking nourishing or indigestible foods
Sleep	• Decrease of night sweats and nycturia, more restful sleep and easier out of bed
Freezing	• Possibility of an increase in freezing due to a decrease in the wrong heat • Possibility of cold feet due to less freezing at the center which finally leads to increasing warmth
Other	• Development of fever ability and healthy sweating • Increasing feeling of coming to oneself and having space for one's self

Improvement is seldom in a straight line. Relapses are part of a good recovery streak. Like a child learning to walk, s/he will fall down often. The under-functioning organs need to learn to "walk" properly.

If we think about the history of tuberculosis, we can easily hypothesize that also in breast cancer supportive treatment strategies may yield further progress. Instead of eradicating the disease, we may be able to help change it from a malignant to a more benign course. This was known when the screening programs were started and distributed. The balance of beneficial and harmful effects of the screening programs and the consequences thereof is judged more negative than positive. Based on this new knowledge, the Swiss Medical Board recommended in 2013 that mammography screening programs should be abolished. The screening programs are a further non-performance of modern medicine to misinterpret every breast cancer cell as a threatening disease and to threaten and burden women with this idea. This has given the consequence of 25-40% over-diagnosed breast cancer patients. Cancer is not necessarily the disease itself if we think of the interaction between disease and host. A healthy host with a well-functioning regeneration has no real or fatal problem with breast cancer. A susceptible host with a weak regeneration, on the other hand, has a real problem. She cannot maintain regeneration and health and avoid death despite all possible eradication therapies. I will now present a case history. Studying the differences in the host and the variability of disease courses, we can use case studies. The RCT, in contrast, is an excellent tool to prove changes and differences, but it can only show average effects. Because of the fact that in our current thinking the host does not matter, we are used to consider statistically idealized average diseases without realizing that this is an academic adulteration of the patient reality. Case studies, in this situation, are the perfect tool to include the host into our attention and to study a classification of the host and of its recovery potential. Careful and sensitive observation makes us aware that diseases, primarily, are an attempt of the body to realize self-healing. In a breast cancer patient of about 50 years of age I have seen that even wide-spread metastases may be such a self-healing attempt. A pathologic fracture of the femur occurred, but in this case, she got high fever a few weeks later and she went to the hospital for care and dying. But the fever appeared to be a healing fever producing painful blisters on the skin. I did not try to order the patient not to die, because Heaven has more power than a doctor. Blisters, incidentally, are taught to be a good sign in ancient Chinese medicine. I just said to the patient that her tongue and pulse looked good, and she should accept that I cannot be God. The only thing was to wait and see what God and destiny is up to. Only a few days after, the wish to die vanished. She wanted to leave the hospital again and to go home. She had an enormous appetite. The only death were her anxieties, and her new courage was seen from the voice that had become firmer. Extensive laboratory and radiological testing showed no more signs of cancer. She was cured and is in good and vital condition until today. It is not always so important how advanced cancer has developed. A resilient host can always recover if host resistance is supported and sufficient. In infectiology and microbiology, the host interaction had long been a fundamental topic. In the modern disease-based thinking, however, even viruses are alleged to be very dangerous. In fact, the first successful vaccination – polio – had made the polio mortality in Berlin disappear, but we usually overlook that infant mortality from all causes remained the same. The undernourished host had remained susceptible to all kinds of infections and total mortality did not change after adoption of the polio vaccination. Thomas McKeown, moreover, showed in 1979 in his study that the decline of infection mortality between 1840 and 1970 (in England and Wales) was considerable, almost linear, before modern medical means were available. The availability of antibiotics and vaccination had no impact on this curve (figure 5).

Figure 5

Thomas McKeown 1979

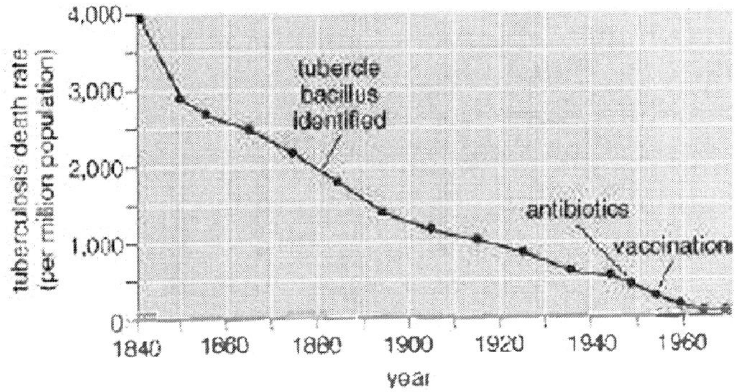

Tuberculosis death rate over 130 years of measurment

McKeown. The role of Medicine: Dream, Miracle or Nemesis? Blackwell, Oxford 1979

It is apparent that innovations in agriculture and housing eliminated starvation and cold and/or damp housing to create this benefit of health and decreased mortality, not medical innovation. Measles occurred in our countries until the seventies – we had measles ourselves as boys. Measles conferred little mortality because we all were well-nourished and well-kept. In third world countries, however, significant measles mortality persisted into the 1980s (i.e. in Nicaragua where I worked as a doctor in a Swiss health brigade). The measles virus was not the cause of severe courses, but malnutrition and lack of schooling. We conducted vaccination programs, but also an agriculture and education reform took place which all together were successful in diminishing measles mortality. We must furthermore assume that the reason for high mortality from the virus of the Spanish flu was deprivation after the world war. A systematic analysis by the Cochrane Collaboration (T Jefferson et al. 2020) showed no effect of influenza vaccination on severe outcomes, even in elderly people. We conclude that immunity is not so much the result of specific antibodies, but mainly of unspecific host resistance not well understood by orthodox medicine. The non-specific host resistance is an urgent topic for medicine to explore. Because we overlook the host interaction, we maintain a false perception of the benefit and necessity of vaccination. Many misunderstandings and errors of preventive medicine have been revealed by evidence-based medicine in the last 25 years. But EBM has been collected by the academic interests of the disease-based specialties. EBM is rather about a thorough critical appraisal of evidence for the individual patient (including his or her number needed to treat and his or her individual diagnostic likelihood of false positive results). What is the prediction for the host in question? Further, we have learned to measure benefit and health by looking at the healthy abilities and overall wellbeing of the patient instead of focusing solely on pathological measures and stages. If medicine is to be beneficial, we must study the host and his or her recovery potential, overcome our irrational fear of death and stop frightening the public and patients with misleading horror statistics.

With this calligraphy (Figure 6) I thank you for your attention.

Figure 6

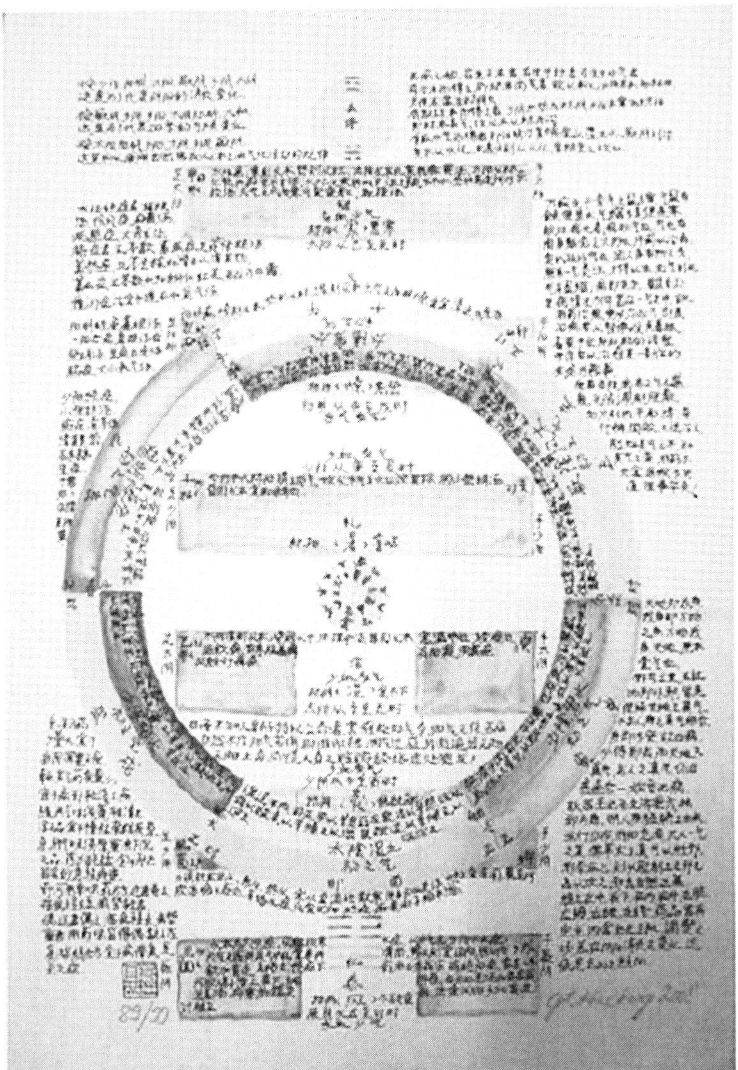

Caligraphic illustration of the universal powers by my teacher Hin Chung Got 2008

Further reading at www.paracelsus-heute.ch.

CHAPTER NINE

BETWEEN DISEASE AND RECOVERY – WHERE AND WHEN IS INTERVENTION OPTIMAL?

Pathology control and disease control as the old medical model is not evidence of a health gain

Speech delivered at the Day of Integrative Medicine, Basel 2014

What is diseased and what is healthy? A simple question – with no simple answer. In medicine today, we orient ourselves to a classification of diseases – to the International Classification of Diseases (ICD). What about a classification of health? We know from practical experience that a healthy digestion, a healthy sleep pattern and care for our strength makes us resilient. We know, but the zeitgeist has taught us to ignore it because medicine believes that healthy functioning of the body's organs does not matter as long as long as diagnostic tests detect pathological findings.

The Swiss academy of medical sciences SAMW believes that one cannot define or specify health and therefore, medicine cannot deal with health. Health would be a philosophical and social issue, but not a medical one.

Do we believe that? Can this be true? Where has medical reasoning got to? Disease findings and abnormal values or test results in healthy persons are considered as evidence of disease. Patients suffering without abnormal findings are considered healthy. Medical reasoning, thus, is trapped in the idea that suffering is the result of pathological findings. Consequently, pathological findings need to be toned down in order to enable health. Medical reasoning believes not only in the error that health is the result of disease elimination but also that elimination of disease creates health. In a very long education doctors learn to view diseases as their enemies and their elimination as his or her heroic acts.

And they learn to see disease-finding as the forerunner of death, and they also learn to frighten people of the many diseases and abnormalities and to yield to sorrow. Most doctors never learn about the rules of medical decision making and to rank their findings accordingly or to ask, "What is the exact benefit for the patient?" Even the SAMW authors get stuck in the grip of such reasoning, though they have written many intelligent thoughts in the paper. It is thus clear that there is little room in conventional medicine for recovery and the ability of the body to self-heal. Self-limiting diseases is indeed a common term, but no-one wants to take the time to wait, the zeitgeist demands immediate activism. The zeitgeist is agitated and hyperactive and gets easily trapped in illusions and false promises and sees spooks behind all the pathological findings. The zeitgeist tends to believe that medicine can eliminate dying, and dying is excluded from everyday life. We cannot overlook that such a zeitgeist determines medical activities more than scientific knowledge.

For about 30 years, however, scientific medicine has developed a measure of health through the school of EBM, which can help us today. The systematic question becomes what constitutes clinical endpoints able to mirror a true patient benefit using abilities and changes or improvements. We can measure the health of a person instead of the degrees of disease which tend to be misleading. Examples are daily living abilities, ability to work, ability to recover or resilience, ability to handle conflict etc. EBM has realized that minimizing a pathology only has a true patient benefit if patient abilities and wellbeing are improved or at least maintained. The degree of disease is less important than the degree of impairment of abilities. This leads us to the awareness that experiential or integrative medicine complies well with EBM. Conventional medicine tends to treat x-rays and laboratory results instead of the patient. Excellent doctors and scientists in conventional medicine have issued a good model 35 years ago (Alvan Feinstein, Clinimetrics, Yale University Press 1987).

In sincere medicine, the question of how to measure health has long been addressed, but it is difficult to penetrate current medical reasoning. The new Swiss Medical Board (SMB), however, also includes ethicists and economists. Conventional medical specialties have followed a model of war on diseases. Contrary to this way of thinking, the SMB has concluded that breast cancer screening and cholesterol screening, for example, are not good for health and should be abolished. 25 years ago, I had the privilege to systematically analyze breast cancer screening and to publish in a well-respected American journal (Schmid, J Clin Epidemiol 1990). The article showed that the alleged benefit of breast cancer screening was a deception. But how could a screening that was able to reduce breast cancer mortality be futile and the benefit be deceptive?

I was sitting in the garden of my Australian beach cottage for many weeks before I could see through it. First, I knew that screening test results may often be false positive. In fact, over 90% of positive mammograms are false positive in the screening context. Second, it had always been the case that breast cancer can also have a benign or malignant course. Therefore, the breast cancer may not be the true problem. Why do some women die from it, but others stay healthy? Do they really die from breast cancer or with breast cancer? Host resistance may be an important determinator which is not known or classifiable by conventional medicine. In fact, autopsy studies show that most breast cancer patients do not become diseased and do not die (Schmidt 1990).

Eventually I understood that the most important question is about how often do beneficial effects occur, and how often do adverse effects occur? This question had not been addressed before I did. This analysis was confirmed by the Cochrane Collaboration 12 years later and by the Swiss Medical Board 25 years later: one woman in 1000 will be prevented from a breast cancer death in 10 years, but she will die from another cause during this time. She will have a 99.9% likelihood that she will not have this luck, but a 15% likelihood that she will have the bad luck of a positive mammogram, and a 1% likelihood that she will be over-diagnosed with the unpleasant treatments that will entail. A woman abstaining from screening may be the 0.1% that will suffer a breast cancer death – instead of death from another cause.

Without screening, women remain healthier. They suffer the same total mortality and avoid unnecessary breast cancer diagnosis and treatment. Medical reasoning promotes such treatment routines that have serious side effects despite such chilling results. The fact that the same cancer has a malignant course in one case, but a benign one in another case in which it does not even get detected during lifetime was intriguing to me and kept me thinking about it. Fear of cancer controls our mind collectively. As doctors, we can be lucky to learn more from courageous patients to see that the true threat is not bad diseases, but fears and prejudice about certain diseases.

The cholesterol story shows erroneous medical reasoning in a similar way. Because there are no healthy and pathological serum cholesterol values, the so-called primary prevention has produced considerable iatrogenic mortality – because cholesterol has been diagnosed and treated, but not the individual human beings. We were made to believe that cholesterol should give us sorrows and distress. If we look at the total mortality figures, however, we can see that one can also die with a normal or treated cholesterol level – in 9 instead of 10 cases in 1000 treatment years, and that one can also survive with a high cholesterol – in 90 instead of 91 cases in 1000 treatment years (Ray et al. Arch Intern Med 2010, Cochrane collaboration 2013) – a healthy body has no real problem with a high cholesterol. A past infarction or a rather rare accumulation of risk factors indicate that there may be a problem with cholesterol, but this is rare. In these situations of very high risk, a cholesterol lowering treatment has a beneficial effect without considering if the cholesterol level is normal or pathological. Modern diseases such as high cholesterol are a misleading artefact of medicine, not a real health problem. Modern society has unlearned to deal productively with death and dying and by doing so, becomes susceptible to false ideas and promises.

Now some Chinese concepts: Breathing into the tan tieng and letting the qi flow – this keeps one healthy. The classical Chinese medicine is analog, not digital. It speaks about the dragon that rises and needs to sink again not to meander in the body and to predicate what can cause disease. Man must be firm below and light and empty in the head – not too top-heavy. And he/she needs a well working center, warm and comfortable and not murky. We should remain in the center, i.e. keep our awareness of the center, to stay healthy.

Now, let's talk about salutogenesis. The five elements in ancient Chinese science are a good model. I found a nice text by a colleague on the internet (www.drhobert.de): I*n the single phases of life we have the energy at our disposal accordingly. In spring, creativity and moxie are at the highest due to the wood energy that will change into the fire energy. Youth and adolescence are the time of expanding activity. Zest for life is at its highest and wants to be satisfied. Growth and discovery, unlimited thinking and acting are determinants of this phase. We hatch out plans and follow our dreams without hesitation. We meet the challenges daily and failure is the reason for new attempts. We are always courageous before conditioning and fears begin to end our readiness for steady growth.*

The following phase of fire is the high point of our courage and desire for trying out new things. The wildfire of love and passion arises. The route to the YOU and to deeper communication open feelings get now reflected. Consciousness becomes broader. Midlife is the change from YANG to YIN. The time of expansion and conquest has come to an end. We now need to focus to our inner life. The onset of the phase of earth leads us to focus to ourselves and our family. We have to give up many things. It is now time for care, loving attention and charity and of new insights through observation and reflection. This change should not be ignored or avoided. Otherwise, the lacking reorientation will result in midlife-crisis. We cannot remain eternally young. Otherwise, gallbladder or heart diseases occur. Birth is not an instant, but a permanent event. Let us consider the saying of ERICH FROMM: "the goal of life is whole and complete birthing. The tragedy is that most of us die before complete birth."

In the fall of life is the time of harvest. Consumption, maturity, wisdom and sense of meaning, awareness and cheerful serenity. Wisdom, understanding, modesty and calm serenity are attributes of the phase of water. Now, life gets accepted as it was. The attitude towards his life may change and result in gratefulness to all what has happened. The readiness to this change is aided by the feeling of having completed everything possible. Everything has its time in life. Like as in archery, we need to release the arrow just in the right moment.
Dr. I. Hobert, Steinhude/Germany

Is myocardial infarction, for example, bad luck or good luck? It may just be the completion of birth and result in a better balance. The observations of my practical work taught me that diseases are often an attempt of the body to restore health. Infarction does not only show a failure in midlife change. It is also a help to pause. A pause can allow new attention to the center. And the pain in the chest draws the attention to the chest and breathing which has had insufficient awareness for a long time. There are many possible disease phenomena which all indicate a change to a better balance and thus a better health for old age. Case stories: Patients under my treatment over a period of 4 years had various illnesses – multiple sclerosis (MS), polyarthritis, colitis, pain diseases, depression and insomnia - all of these symptoms can aid a change to allow recovery. One example will illustrate this notion. I am treating a singer now for 2 ½ years because of migraine, backpain, psoriasis and fatigue for many years. She also has nycturia and freezing hands, feet and nose. The symptoms were caused by an unbalance of the liver – center – lung axis with extensive cold due to Yang deficiency. Especially the center was deficient. The digestion was weak and unable to clear. The turbidity goes to the skin. Hypermenorrhea and lack of mental balance also confirm the weakness in the center. After two years of herbal treatment to strengthen spleen Yang, much had improved such as the migraine, the skin, sleep, backache, freezing and digestion. A stronger center also means more inner calm. Meanwhile, the patient complained of indifference that was more than before. I looked at her and examined her face and asked: how is singing? Better and better, she said, her voice had become more expressive again. We can see that it was a healthy indifference which she did not like. Liveliness is not the same as restlessness and hyperactivity. We need a sound understanding of what is healthy.

If we look at MS, we should understand that the number of attacks is of minor importance. Attacks are the natural attempt of the body to clear pathogenic factors such as cold and dampness as we call it in classical Chinese medicine. An indication of this damp and cold is a longstanding pale and swollen tongue. The outbreak of MS, thus, is a healthy clearing attempt of the body to recover, although damp and cold may impair peripheral nerves for a long time. Cold leads to false heat and/or inflammation. Dampness anaesthetizes and causes numbness. But the vital center gets discharged and can function properly again which is important to maintain the strength and future health. In many cases, patients recover from attacks because the body becomes capable of clearing the pathogenic factors also from the peripheral extremities and to complete the clearing process. In some cases, MS has quite a benign course leading to spontaneous recovery. In other cases, the course is rather malignant and can even lead to death. If we understand that treating and strengthening the host may make the difference, we do not need to treat the disease because the host makes the disease alter from a malignant to a benign course and outcome. Attacks are a sign that the host is still competent to initiate a healthy clearing process. Attacks are a promising sign of resilience. Therefore, the suppression of attacks with interferon etc. is Pyrrhus medicine. Indeed, side effects of interferon are influenza-like syndromes, anorexia, digestive disorder, insomnia and headache which all are signs of cold pathogens. Interferon blocks the body's ability to react with healthy clearing maneuvers. This may promote bad outcomes in the end. Indeed, the Cochrane collaboration concludes that the available interferon trials are not qualified to show a clear benefit to the patients. A case history: a 29-year-old woman had been under my treatment for 4 years. At the age of 23, the first attack occurred. She experienced numbness of her fingers and a vision disorder. The history revealed premature birth and cold hands and feet for many years. She needs socks in bed to keep her feet warm, and she had nycturia as a child. She dislikes winter and prefers summer. She has impaired sweating but fever only once at the age of 10 with fancy dreams. She often had otitis media, back ache and a lumbago attack at age 20. Her stool was often loose, and she was ravenous. She slept poorly as a child with nightmares. She often slept in the bed together with her parents. Her menstruation was irregular and scarce. She had low blood pressure with dizziness. Her tongue was pale and swollen with teeth marks, but her pulse showed some power. There was a good precondition as her senses were adequate and favorable. She protects herself from cold and does not permanently seek cold to cool the false heat of inflammation as it is often seen. For understanding the situation, it is important to see that the MS symptoms are of secondary importance. They are a healing phenomenon. The overall strength and resilience are of primary importance. This allows improvement of digestion and freezing as well as normal sweating and the ability to develop fever. This is needed for the elimination of cold. When the pathogenic damp and cold diminish, the nerve lesions can recover. I prescribed a cold formula for many months that eliminates cold and to build and maintain Yang and to allow sweating and to increase blood flow. I told her not to give blood for diagnostic purposes and to keep her feet warm all the time. Nutrition should deliver a lot of Yang. Eating meat, especially lamb, chicken, beef and game and prawns is favorable as well as long cooking broth. In summer 2012, the patient had normal sweating without a red head. Her feet were warm, and she had less sense of cold. Her stool had become normal, and she had a good appetite without ravenousness. She lost some weight, and her tongue became less pale, but not yet optimal. Due to the hot weather in August 2012, she had another attack with numbness of the lower body. One night she also had bladder dysfunction, but her sleep became much better which indicates that cold had emigrated from the center. Her weight loss together with a healthy appetite occurred because the damp and cold had left the body. She became more courageous and confident and overcame the short shock of being frightened by neurological indoctrination. After 2 months of therapy, all numbness and paresthesia disappeared and this persisted until today. This shows that attacks are a healing process important for the good outcome. She perceived that the old-fashioned nutrition did her good. In contrast she realized that vitamin and power drinks which were recommended to her by others did not do her good, they are Yin and powerless. Let's come back to the question in the title: when and where is the optimal intervention?

Should we have used steroids during her last attack to minimize symptoms? It was obviously not necessary as we could see. However, we may improve Yang and the capacity of natural healing processes as well as suppressing symptoms. The problem is that steroids bring additional cold to the body and increases the precarious susceptibility. The process of recovery is often a path on a ridge, which makes rigid rules counterproductive. The intuition and sensitivity of the doctor is more important to see what is needed. The perception of the patient is a great help that can be used. Each patient needs another herbal formula that fits to his or her power architecture, but the same formula can be used for similar patients with different diseases – the formula for a patient with e.g. pollinosis, polyarthritis, lumbago or insomnia could be the same. The condition of the heart, which is considered the emperor of all organs, determines to what extent a person is astute and has a balanced perception of things. If a man unable to swim, for example, falls into the water, he has the chance to quickly learn to swim and to save himself. It does not really matter if he had fallen by accident or if he had been pushed into the water. The pushed one may seek help from outside – and lose time. The hearty spirit makes the difference and determines the adequate perception and confers the ability to see the chance, or only dark if the spirit is not hearty. A man who does not see heartily uses his power wrongly and exhausts it. Through a disease he can detect his hearty spirit. It is always important for a man to become his own doctor and to see that he cannot live against the power he has.

We now can define health as healthy reaction of the body to damage and stress, thus as an intact recovery potential which includes healthy sleep, healthy digestion, healthy inner warmth, healthy grieving, healthy depression, healthy indifference and listlessness etc. Also dying is part of a good health.

Where is intervention optimal?

We have demonstrated that the conventional nosology and ICD does not allow a diagnosing of the patient situation. One patient can die from a certain disease, but another may have only light problems. Conventional medicine treats both the same. Conventional medicine is harmful if it does not understand that current diagnoses are insufficient. We need a diagnosis of the patient in addition, and of his individual recovery potential. Optimal intervention needs a more profound understanding of the interaction between pathogenesis and salutogenesis.

To summarize: Study natural recovery and publish your knowledge about it. As practitioners of integrative medicine, you are in a privileged position. We wish you success in this endeavor.

CHAPTER TEN

SCIENTIFIC EVIDENCE, THE PATIENT AND THE ART OF MEDICINE

First published in Primary Care EMH Basel 2014
http://www.paracelsus-heute.ch/cms/literatur/PDF/PrimaryCare2014.pdf

Also today, the art of medicine remains a topical issue

There are few conditions in which there are specific treatments for specific diseases [1]. It is a strange connudrum that every human being is an individual unlike any other, even in the case of so-called identical twins, and yet hospital systems routinely and doggedly attempt to standardize treatment regimes. In practice, we are faced with different, indiviudal patients. Their overall picture is determined by the interplay of pathogenesis (the background and challenge to the health of the patient) and salutogenesis (the ability of the patient to fight off the challenge) – by the disease and the recovery potential of the patient/host. Diseases are always compensated to some extent by self-healing and resilience, and in some cases even surmounted. Supportive measures which focus on the patient resilience and his/her overall health can change a bad course into a favorable one, without the necessity of treating the disease with the tools with have at our disposal. The mission of medicine has always been to treat whatever whatever aflictted the patient with the tools at our disposal and not only his/her symptoms. Meticulous diagnostic work-ups utilizing traditional laboratory and picture diagnostic methods as well as treatments of the diseases with insuffincinet attention to side effects and interactions often harm the patient rather than benefit him/her.

Variability and complexity of the patient situation

It calls for greater skepticism when olserving the current use of statistical methods which all too often overshadow the study object itself. The background for such overkill is all to often to make shabby research look good and to smooth the great variability in individuals that disturbs academic routine. The father of the modern double blind randomized controlled trial (dubbed DBRCT) Dr. Alvin Feinstein, who besides being a world renowned researcher, was himself an astute, fine feeling physician able to asuage and help his patients. In his seminal book Clinimetrics, he devoted a chapter to the common traps of DBRCTs and why the randomized patient was never represetative of the real patient at a busy hospital ward where there was no time to dilly dally.

The great natural aberrations are all too obvious in the practice of medicine. Years of professional experience lead to new insights that teach us to see the recovery potential of the patients and teaches us to take seriously the views and beliefs of the patients which is essential in the overall diagnosis. Some patients know better than doctors their path to health – even if the path looks risky. Recovery knows that "All roads lead to Rome".

We should always have the benefit of the individual patient foremost in our deliberations. Then we can use our experience and differentiated knowledge of human nature as well as a solid basis in scientific evidence to make the best therapy available to him/her. Evidence from DBRCTs is the best we have. However, such studies constitute an average finding and the number needed to treat is usually so large that an effective treatment is difficult to ascertain in the individual case. Futhermore, the pleuripharamceutical patient has many side effects and interactions that can, despite the findings from the DBRCT, lead to a bad result. On the other hand, the outcome can be good. We always need to bear in mind the 2x2 table and the many deviations from the mean (fig. 1). This table illustrates that there are always a number of patients suffering disadvantages and harm from a treatment that is effective and beneficial on average. On the basis of the diagnosis alone, we are often unable to predict if the treatment or non-treatment will lead to a favourable or unfavourable outcome in our individual patient. We must constantly question the treatment – will it truly help our patient or produce adverse effects. We are faced with the question of whether we can identify the patients who will benefit or be harmed by the treatment singled out in the DBRCT. Does the drug support or strain or weaken the patient? In a sensitive medical practice, we see that the opinion and attitude of the patient, and his/her way of thinking and hoping, play an important role. Our facilitator role can instigate the activism, but we should not exert pressure on the patient. The decision for treatment can always be right or wrong as can the decision against treatment. Futhermore, effective diagnostics can be right or wrong, and confer benefit or harm [4].

Figure 1.

	Disease				
Test	True positive	a	c	False positive	Test positive
	False negative	b	d	True negative	Test negative
	Diseased			Healthy	

Sensitivity = $a/a+c$

Specificity = $d/b+d$

Positive predictive value (PPD) = $a/a+b$

Negative predictive value (NPD) = $d/c+d$

Prevalence = $a+b/a+b+c+d$

EBM

In medicine, formal scientific evidence offers only vague or incomplete knowledge. This is due to the fact that science cannot take into account the notion of indivduality that is central to any sensitive medical practice. The notion of evidence-based treatments represents false scholastic overinterpretation, keeping in mind that every patient is an individual unlike any other and is prone to react differently than the average. Evidence-based therapies are an option which can be chosen or not, especially if the patient is not happy with it or adverse effects make it unpleasant. The doctor might have other options which are well thought out, for example light therapy (see chapters 3 and 4). Many results from controlled trials are substiantal, but they cannot tell us how we best can treat our individual patient. The historic achievement of the controlled trial is its potential to identify medical errors such as *confounding bias* and *surrogate fallacies*. EBM sidesteps these issues by utilizing state of the art epidemiological tools and suspecting falacies at every turn.

References

1 See chapter 4.
2 L. Litschgi, Primary care 2012, EMH Basel 2012.
3 See chapter 3.
4 J. Schmidt. in M.M. Kochen editor. Allgemein- und Familienmedizin. Thieme, Stuttgart 2006.
5 JG Schmidt, Eur J Gen Practice 1999.
6 JG Schmidt. Placebo. Forsch. Komplementärmed. 1998. Karger Basel.
7 AR Feinstein. *in* Schmidt JG and Steele RE. Kirchheim Verlag, Mainz 1994.
8 JG Schmidt. Patients with Multiple Sclerosis. Swiss J for Holistic Medicine. Karger Basel 2013.

CHAPTER ELEVEN

PRINCIPLES OF EFFECTIVE REHABILITATION MEDICINE

My own experience in a misguided rehabilitation clinic is still quite fresh.

Observations and Findings

These observations are the result of my personal experience, together with the analytical tools of clinical epidemiology and EBM. Medical science has experienced significant changes in the last decades. The criteria for treatment success have dramatically changed (see chapter 1). However, subjects such as immunology, obstetrics/gynecology and neurology are reluctant to adopt these changes. In specialized neurological clinics the error prevails that the clinic would carry out the rehabilitation. This is of course utterly wrong because it is the patient himself who carries out the rehabilitation. The role of the clinic is to support and not to hinder him. The deplorable habit of establishing long lists of diagnoses and to treat the single diagnoses separately – therapy of the feet, of the legs, the upper extremities and the brain – is not very effective in practice. The patient is 1 person that cannot be divided without harm. I had my first hemiplegia. At that time, I was in a clinic in the mountains near heaven/sky. The personnel heard what I wanted and let me do things at my own discretion. After only a few weeks I was able to return home to my work as a doctor. The conventional reduction of disease parameters and pathological findings is not always a benefit to patients. However, I landed in a clinic in Eastern Thurgau which earlier had been a psychiatric clinic. The hostile and overprotecting spirit towards the patients was still oozing out of the walls and bedazzled the staff. Effective rehabilitation could start only after leaving the clinic. I then married a female farmer in Thailand and helped her as much as possible doing the farm work. In winter, we usually live in Thailand and spend the summer in Switzerland. The rehabilitation became truly effective only after the Swiss social authorities (KESB) bowed out.

On the farm we have coconut trees, bananas, pineapples, and figs, buffalo, pigs and chickens. Rehabilitation is more effective at home because the clinics do not treat the one person, but the single diagnosis. At least at clinic Z in the old psychiatry building, the pseudo-professional approach was practiced by the staff. The suggestions of the patient were devalued as trivial and dismissed. Only qigong and bladder rehabilitation by Prof. Hohlbrugger and Mrs. Branz showed a true beneficial effect in this leading clinic Z.

Moreover, the dogma of the last century that damaged brain cannot recover, seems still to prevail among neurologists. Conventional clinics determine the goals of their patients, and medical prognoses are notoriously prone to error. Most doctors have no idea about false negative and false positive test results and of the danger of overdiagnosis. One episode can illustrate the fallacy of the common disease-based reasoning. While in the rehab clinic I had a fall in the toilet with no injury. Instead of recognizing my ability to react instinctively to avoid injury, however, the doctor misdiagnosed the fall as a sign of brain damage. She was a typical representative of the common misconception of disease-based thinking and could not see my will power of recovery and being healthy. But I had many crashes* and even near-drownings** in my life with no bad or fatal injury. It is not my merit, but a gift from Heaven, and it is important to be considered by a doctor.

If one views the many reports about successful recovery, it becomes evident that commitment and individualism of the patient are important predictors of good recovery, even if the patient makes risky decisions in the eyes of the doctor. The GP Litschgi of Basel has therefore suggested the patient should be the driver and the doctor the passenger.

*At the age of 2, I crawled from underneath a car which had run over me.
**In the Atlantic Ocean, I was about to drown when I suddenly got very calm and realized that I could let the waves spit me out onto the beach.

My neurological abilities had a long history that the doctor ignored.

I. Consequences And Principles

A. Patient is the Driver; the doctor is passenger.

This suggestion of Litschgi would be important for the entire medical practice, but especially important in rehabilitation medicine. The determination of goals based on medical prognoses should be considered an error.

B. Daily Life Relevance
In one's own home rehabilitation is more effective than in specialized clinics. Clinics not following these principles should be closed. Old age and nursing homes may be a better and more economical alternative.

C. **No need for expensive robots.** There seems to be a tendency to use expensive robots to enhance a perception of quality. This cannot compensate for a lack of the other quality principles.

D. **Ambitious goals and plenty of time.** As written in other parts of this text, one must be patient. Very often, time makes all the difference.

E. **Rehabilitation** is a life-long learning process which reflects life as such. New goals are helpful, but time pressure and deadlines are not helpful.

CHAPTER TWELVE

A NOVEL AND EFFECTIVE TREATMENT MODALITY FOR MEDICALLY UNEXPLAINED SYMPTOMS

RICHARD EVAN STEELE, EVELYNE DE LEEUW AND DAVID O. CARPENTER

Abstract: Medically unexplained symptoms (MUS) confound physicians, and the incidence and prevalence of these conditions is poorly documented. This is not least due to the complex nature of MUS and mimicry of morbidity with conditions that have common clinical assessment and treatment modalities, e.g. migraine headaches which stress headaches commonly are misdiagnosed as. Effective treatment modalities for MUS have been more or less non-existent. In the following we present a modality for the assessment, diagnosis and treatment of MUS that in our experience leads to cure, at least in better than half of these cases measured in terms of allowing the individual *back to work*. These results are at least twice as high as those described hitherto (see below), and yet, our treatment modality is beset with many obstacles, not the least of which is the intransigence of a system that will not and/or can not understand why this modality is so much better than what they are able to offer. The most important obstacle is financing, as this modality requires long term and committed financing to work. The economic implications of not dealing with these issues are described.

Keywords: medically unexplained symptoms, back to work

Background

For decades authors have described, in varying levels of detail, classification, quantification and assessment of the economic impact of patients with medically unexplained symptoms (MUS) [1, 2]. The syndromes commonly presenting to clinicians lacking discernable and/or measurable, concrete symptoms include, but are no means limited to, whiplash syndrome, chronic fatigue syndrome, post-viral syndrome, chronic lower back pain, chronic stress headache, chronic muscle pain and various others. More recently a few studies have surfaced which assess various treatment modalities for this group, and the conclusion until now has been disappointing. In what we view as the best review of the area to date it is clearly stated that there is no effective treatment modality for this group [3, 4, 5]. In all of the cited works, a commendable effort to adhere to the standardized approach to treatment evaluation is applied. We present a novel approach which departs significantly from previous attempts in five delineable areas, namely how the patients are triaged, where the treatment takes place, who delivers the treatment, how the treatment is individualized and what the dependent variable is for evaluation of the treatment. We have demonstrated that the described treatment modality can bring better than half of the patients treated from a generally painful and disabled state back to the workforce, and that the methodology of the modality is generalizable.

In dealing with MUS patients, it is imperative to dare to leave the world of the double blind, randomized and controlled trial (DBRCT) behind. This is predicated by the highly individual circumstances leading to MUS and the enormous variation in the response type to these circumstances. This variation is highly dependent on many personal psychological traits, perhaps the most important of which is resiliency, which is at best a difficultly quantifiable trait [6]. Even in the best of the DBRCT world, the issue of patient variation and the lack of congruence between the standardized trial person and the real-world use of the intervention and/or medication in question is problematical. The father of clinimetrics, the late Alvin Feinstein, discusses this problem at length in the seminal volume Clinimetrics [7, 8]. The issue is clearly evident to the practicing physician who is seldom able to directly correlate the patient model in the typical DBRCT trial to his/her daily round patients (if indeed he/she even attempts to assess this) nor is able to apply the conclusions drawn from the typical DBRCT directly to the practical clinical situation. In the typical MUS patient (given this term makes any sense at all given the above), these problems become all the more critical precisely because the issues leading to MUS are highly individual and therefore impossible to match. Further, the typical MUS patient would refuse to participate in a study that involved a treatment modality that for example tested the efficacy of delivering treatment locally versus her having to travel with her symptoms to a centralized unit delivering the same service. Why would a chronic pain patient participate in a trial of this nature and risk having to go through many painful journeys when the expertise can be delivered locally? Further, why would a chronic pain patient expect a good result from a standardized approach when an individualized approach is offered? Taking this logic one step further, when it is obvious (to the patient, at least) that delivering this sort of treatment locally and individually tailored is better than a painful journey for the patient to and from a centralized unit to a standardized treatment, how would one defend allocating one patient to a local and individualized offer and thereby force the "match" to go through the normal pattern of a centralized unit? Further yet, if this treatment modality is so obviously superior to the centralized offer, what use is a study of any nature (excluding of course an evaluation of the efficacy)?

In the world of the stringent DBRCT the methodological issues often overshadow the item of study, i.e. statistical evaluations of survey tools or detailed descriptions of the matching and/or randomization process, but these issues are rarely candidly discussed by the authors in terms of issues of validity and reliability. This lack of self-critical discussion is widely accepted in scientific journals, for which reason these have a decided tendency to favor DBRCT studies over treatises that call this practice into question [9]. This so-called evidence-based world will invariably miss the most important parts of the story behind MUS exactly because one can not put together a trial which standardizes the patient with psychological trauma and the individual responses thereto that fuel MUS [10] for the reasons just mentioned. The resistance to this argumentation which invariably will come forth from the DBRCT powers is not, we argue, a weakness in our reasoning, but rather a weakness in the DBRCT model. Let them show better results with this group, and we will let our arguments fall. This is discussed at greater length below.

Review protocols by the internationally esteemed Cochrane Collaboration have traditionally emphasized the value of experimental designs in the generation of evidence [11]. However, as Sir Archibald Cochrane states himself as a key principle in his foundational work, evidence can only be generated *with* patients, not on patients. This principle is now increasingly recognized, the vanguard of a multi-methodological approach being led by the Cochrane Health Promotion and Public Health Field [12]. This initiative emphasizes the necessity of gathering all kinds of evidence, not just the “hard” evidence gathered by the typical DBRCT comparing one medical intervention to the other, or against placebo.

The kind of thinking necessary here is how to create evidence that setting a broken bone is better than not setting it. This has never been the issue of a DBRCT, yet no one questions it. Designing a DBRCT for the purpose of finding whether setting a bone is effective would be highly nonsensical as well as unethical. The same kind of logic applies to the treatment modality presented here, and the same level of nonsense and unethicality applies to the issue of creating a trial that shows the difference.

This does not mean that anything goes, however. In our experience, quality and the fundability of a given treatment modality which can not be tested is dependent on clear outcome measures that make sense to all involved (e.g. setting a broken bone). In dealing with MUS patients, our outcome variable is *back to work* – short but sweet. We maintain that the re-engagement of the MUS patient in the work force is the strongest statement that can be made regarding the quality of the treatment modality. In our view, this output variable is just as strong as the healing of a broken bone. In addition to this dependent variable, certain basic elements of what constitutes a reasonable and fundable activity must be maintained (see below).

The economic impact of MUS is widely recognized as being enormous, and growing [13, 14]. The discourse around the socio-economic impact of MUS is, we maintain, nevertheless unfocused and often obscure. The most important issue in this context is that there is no standardized registration of this group as such, and how would one devise such a registration? As noted above, MUS patients are seen by various specialists because of symptoms that mimic commonly assessable and treatable disease entities [15]. As long as the specialists in question have yet to rule out the typical symptomology they are used to, the MUS patient remains undiagnosed. Meanwhile, MUS is not a recognized disease entity and there is no consensus as to what sort of specialist is relevant in these cases. For this reason among others, the majority of MUS patients are unseen by appropriate assessment experts. This compounds the difficulty in quantifying MUS. In Denmark, where this experience comes from, doctors are, mostly for the better, an integral cog in the bureaucracy of social welfare and health care, i.e. they play an important role in decisions regarding social welfare for unable and/or disabled individuals. The primary author has spent more than five years functioning as a medical consultant for a series of Danish communities. Approx. 10,000 sick leave patient dossiers were reviewed by him during this period. It is important to mention that for at least half of these cases, the work up and conclusions regarding the described condition were perfectly clear and problem free. The other approximately half of this cohort had, however, not been given relevant or appropriate assessment, diagnosis or care – they demonstrated issues that were not described or dealt with relevantly at earlier stages of the disabling process. An example will elucidate the how and why of this problem.

A 35-year-old male presents with severe lower back pains after a lifting trauma at his workplace some days earlier. The physician finds no dermatomical issues but only muscle tenderness and orders some days' rest and a standard NSAID medicine prescription. Some weeks later, the GP is approached by the community to deliver a physician's note that the patient is not work ready. The GP calls in the patient, and he now has radial pains minding the GP of a slipped disc. The GP refers to the specialist route, and 4 months later there is an MR scan that shows clearly that there is no pathology in and/or surrounding the spinal column that can explain the patient's symptoms. During the ensuing months, the social system fails to catch the MUS in this case, and first when the primary author is presented with the case after this period is the suspicion aroused that there is something here that does not add up. Through interviewing and document mining, it turns out that the patient is dyslectic, passed his grade school with no referral to this phenomenon, could not do his basic arithmetic nor read as evidenced by the tests set in motion by the primary author. Refusing to take these issues into account and deal with them, the community awarded the patient a permanent disability pension based on his inability to work and the conclusion by all of the specialists (save the primary author) that the man was untreatable. The man is intelligent enough to realize where his shortcomings are, and this awareness has led to one experienced failure after the other until he no longer was able to handle the constant reminding of all which he could not do. This led to what can be likened to an early mid-life crisis which led to poor sleep habits and a generally tense muscle state that again led to chronic muscle tenderness which explains why the relatively light trauma in the story predicated the full-blown pain syndrome that he ended up with.

Would this development have been avoidable? Obviously. The first step that falters is of course the parents and the school where the patient attended. They failed to address in time that the described individual was going to leaving school with a reasonable modicum of what is needed to participate in a modern workforce. The next level of what goes wrong has to do the workplace per se, because the only work generally available to this type of young man is hard menial labor. The fact that hard menial labor tends to lead to early disability is extremely well documented [16, 17]. The negative effects of hard menial labor are often compounded by untoward conditions at workplaces of this nature, including insufficient machines and tools for lifting, poor ventilation and monotonous, routine work.

Is this man treatable? Definitely. See more below.

The assessment that serious issues in the case described and the many thousands like it have not been uncovered during the disease generating process is based on the simple fact that these patients were in a more debilitated state than the description of their case could explain (n = approx. 5000). This is not based on a concrete assessment using validated tools, but rather the "best man's best opinion". We maintain that nothing better is available, and that this evaluation is good enough, given the enormous lack of relevant treatment modalities for the individuals in question. Given an average proportion of the population on sick leave at 7% in Denmark, this equivalates to roughly 3.5% of the population with some or other degree of MUS. Officially, there were in May 2005 157,000 persons in Denmark, or roughly 3% of the population, in social grouping levels 4 and 5, which in Denmark means that the person in question has work disability beyond what can be dealt with through standard work force related activities [18]. The official and our observed percentages given here correlate well, but as described above, there is no hard data to corroborate this. This is not so important, however. Any epidemiological assessment has its uncertainties, and it makes little difference if the real figure is 2%, 3,5% or 5%. The problems for the individual patient and the cost to society are still completely unacceptable.

Given one accepts the prevalence estimate as reasonable, and that the figure is more or less uniform in countries with similar socio-economic conditions, it is relatively simple to extrapolate the yearly cost of disability pay and other costs for these patients, not the least of which is irrelevant usage of primary, secondary, tertiary and alternative health care and other resources. The following figures may help the reader. The support level and a rough estimate of health care usage for a Danish MUS patient is the equivalent of EUR 2500 per month. Assuming that this patient does not return to the workforce, that the age of MUS onset is 35 years, and that the old age pension begins at age 67, then the discounted outlay from society in 2007 EUR is 2,360,000 (standard forward value calculation utilizing a 5% interest rate). Depending on the national tax level, this figure is roughly from 30% to 50% too low, as it does not take lost tax revenue into account. The interesting facet of this exercise is twofold: it elucidates the economic impact of MUS, and it puts into perspective that the cost of treatment of such cases is less interesting than whether it works. If the average cost of treatment is EUR 35,000, and the success rate is 50%, then the return on investing in treatment is a staggering 3300% over 31 years (still assuming age of MUS onset 35 years and an average time of treatment one year). As anyone familiar with investment thinking will attest, not investing in effective treatment of MUS patients is tantamount to financial suicide. Multiplying these figures by the total number of MUS patients worldwide gives figures that defy the imagination. As stated above, the real figures are unavailable, but they are also not so important. The logic presented here fails to impress most politicians, as they tend to see only the cost of treatment, and either fail or refuse to grasp the long-term advantages. This is one of the obstacles mentioned in the beginning of this article.

As stated above, very few published works show success in the treatment of this group of patients, and none of these have demonstrated the level of success we present here. The literature is almost wholly limited to the description of the group. There are numerous weaknesses in this work, the most serious of which is the lack of specificity and sensitivity of the instruments used. We maintain that this is an inherent flaw in nearly all clinical evaluations which is sorely accentuated in the MUS population. In the cited literature, the undescribed characteristics of the individual patient are a serious source of confounding. In our experience, the typical (see above) MUS patient has strong personal and individually unique experiences and characteristics that make grouping and categorizing useless at best, and counterproductive or even dangerous for the patient at worst [19]. Besides the drug issues cited, this observation comes from the experience of the primary author as medical consultant and as clinical chief of the treatment modality described here, with N = 134 to date (number of patients examined).

Recruitment of patients

Patient recruitment for the group described in this publication has not been via a defined study nor through a clear clinical channel, e.g. referral to a cardiologist for chest pains and an abnormal ECG. The patients that are described here are all fringe patients with serious pain and/or psychological problems that every other clinical entity that exists in Denmark has defined as beyond clinical reach, i.e. the clinic in question has no treatment to offer. As such, patient recruitment has followed a pattern of being the treatment of last resort for patients that have no other modalities available. Patients found us through word of mouth or by being described as needing the treatment modality described by the primary author in his function as medical consultant. The small number of patients described here in general and the even smaller number of those that have completed treatment is a reflection of the severe difficulty in getting payers of health care to understand how and why so much more can be done for these patients if one is willing and able to go the distance in long term care delivered locally and the implementation of the interprofessionality necessary for positive movement in the patient condition. That we have any results to publish at all is due to the largesse of a few Danish communities and a short period (9 months) during which we had a financing agreement with the Danish central hospital authority. This agreement was undermined by several factors, the most important of which is the same system intransigence to change that is touched upon above, despite the logic presented here. Other issues weighed in, among these the fact that the clinicians set to evaluate our reports had not the clinical knowledge necessary to do so, but that is another issue sorely in need of development and a book or two on the subject. As of this writing, the clinic has ceased to function due to lack of a workable financial model.

Methods

The following sections of this article describe in some detail the examination and treatment of the MUS patient. Further information is available through contact with the primary author.

Patient examination

The examination is crucial to uncovering at least the main facets of the syndrome presented. No single exam can uncover all aspects of the syndrome for the simple reason that time does not allow this. Furthermore, the psychological genesis of the syndrome very often has elements that only come out when the patient is ready to report it. An example will elucidate this. Patient NN presents with a pain syndrome which starts with a modest trauma to the left knee during a roller-skating incident when she was 12 years old. The patient developed an untoward movement pattern based on persistent pains in her left knee. Over the 20 years that pass until we meet her, she has developed chronic pains in her back, the left hip and thigh as well as stomach pains tied to defecation problems. From the start, the symptoms did not reflect a common causality, and with time, the patient confided in us that she had experienced what in positive terms could be called bestial sexual habits forced on her by a psychotic "lover". The point is not only that this case begs for the kind of help we can offer, but that each patient has her personal experience that condition the syndrome that ensues, and that this individuality precludes a standardized treatment approach. It makes no sense to rubricize this patient as having been through deviant sexual abuse, because no two patients so rubricized will have experienced enough of the same to warrant a standardized approach to treatment. Further, individual resiliency is sufficiently variable that some women will sublimate such experiences and be OK notwithstanding, and others will have varying levels of debilitating to extremely debilitating reactions thereto. This variability conditions an individual approach to the patient which a standardized modality is unable to carry out.

This being said, it is clear that the approach to the patient needs to be interprofessional, since no one individual health professional can cover the breadth of needed therapies and examinations to help and/or cure the patient. The patient described and all of her co-patients have various degrees of combined psychological and somatic symptoms that are closely tied to each other yet very difficult to approach due to the general phenomenon among these patients that they have accustomed themselves to their condition. They have their syndrome as part of their daily life and therefore part of their identity. Further, they are used to and have accepted the conclusions given that there is no treatment available. This altered identity can not be challenged without a reaction from the patient which in many cases presents a serious challenge for the interprofessional team. We have experienced several patients that simply would not put up with this challenge. We were forced to concede failure from the start, as these patients appear to be completely uninterested in improving [20]. To our knowledge, no systematical knowledge regarding this phenomenon (i.e.

not wanting to get better) exists, although the issue is tangent to the neuroses of psychiatry.

More specifically and generally, the exam follows a reasonably common template:

The work-up of the treatment modality has to date been carried out by the primary author and a psychologist trained in pain assessment and cognitive therapy.

- The work-up starts with introductions and presentation of credentials for staff and patient. The process establishes the necessary decor and professionalism of the event, avoiding the risk of undue familiarity as well as ensuring reasonable cooperation ("we are here to help you, and we are qualified to do so").
- Then we conduct a semi-structured interview. The interview varies much partly due to previous knowledge of the patient (other work-ups prior to our examination which we of course study prior to the exam when such is available) and the course of events in the individual patient history. Areas always covered include the full spectrum of patient life and health experience as much as patient memory allows. We cover birth and childhood, schooling, early adulthood and adulthood to date with full disclosure of relationships to spouse, parents, siblings, schoolmates and other relevant persons/institutions.
- Patient income, social relations and work history are covered. Special emphasis is placed on psychological health spanning life to date, and how this is correlated to employment or lack thereof.

This process takes up an hour to 1½ hours of interview time during which we in all but a few cases to date reach a level of empathy and trust with the patient that motivates her to reveal things that are deep secrets that few if any have ever heard before. This is partly due to our interview technique, which is highly culturally sensitive and patient centered (this also works through an interpreter), and partly due to the highly unusual situation the patient finds him or herself in, spending around two hours with what for most of them is the first physician to take their complaints seriously.
After the semi-structured interview, a structured interview regarding health issues is conducted, covering the usual sum of medically relevant issues: disposition, allergies, organ symptoms (including sexual health), medications, substance abuse, tobacco and alcohol use. The work-up then

moves on to a full physical examination utilizing a mobile gurney that is carried along to every exam as well as the normal array of medical tools including stethoscope, opthalmo/otoscope, blood pressure device, light source, tongue depressor, cotton swabs and reflex hammer.

During the work-up the physician and the psychologist supplement each other, take over the interview, tease a comment apart, fill in blanks, explain the odd misunderstanding and reassure the patient when one or the other oversteps a psychological threshold. In most cases, this leads to several outbursts of joviality, which increases patient empathy. The work-up gives the patient reassurance that the team is up to what if offers. All through the work-up, both the physician and the psychologist observe the patient – his/her movements, length of composure in one or more positions, facial expressions, emotional response range, normal, quasi-normal or abnormal behavior and responses and of course reactions to given instructions during the physical exam.

At the conclusion of the work-up, we explain our findings and the treatment strategy we envisage. We have not to date met any patients that did not accept our offer with two exceptions. These patients were brought to us by social authorities more or less against their will. In both cases we quickly discerned that the patients were neither interested in treatment nor in confiding their case to us, as discussed above.

Once we have our work-up back from the secretary, it is proof read and then sent on to the referring physician (clinical chief of one of the public clinics treating MUS patients) who evaluates the work-up and either gives it a go ahead or the opposite. This is highly problematical in that the referring physicians are generally not attuned to the psychosocial aspects of the case and therefore tend to view our work-ups as insufficiently medical to warrant the green light for treatment to begin. Thus, a little more than half of the patients we have evaluated have not been treated. Attempts to turn this behemoth around have fallen to the ground so far and for reasons unknown to us, both the medical press and the daily press have been unwilling to take this serious problem up. We can only speculate that the failure to integrate our procedures into mainstream medical practice and media is due to the fact that our approach challenges the current medical-professional paradigm – if not "evidence based", it can not be good.

In those cases where treatment (financing) is approved, it is instigated. Initially, emphasis is on creating trust and getting a fuller picture of the background for MUS, which normally is described during the work-up but rarely fully enough to allow a full picture of the therapeutic effort.

Treatment

The novelty of this treatment modality is fivefold:

1) Triage of the patient adheres to the principles outlined above. We assume that the patient has issues that are not described and delve into these issues during the primary exam. This requires a physician highly attuned to MUS and able to tease typical somatic problems and psychosomatic problems apart. The psychologist supports this and together the triage leads to the relevant treatment plan;

2) Treatment is delivered in the patient's home or very close to there. There are 4 very good reasons for this:

    a) the patient avoids the transport to and from the centralized service. For most patients, this is not an insurmountable obstacle, but for the chronic pain patient, the time and untoward seating in transport take more away from the treatment than can be given at the centralized unit,

    b) after the session, the patient can sit back and relax instead of having to enter the transport home. The value of this is great, as most of our sessions leave the patient with heavy thinking to do and/or a deep relaxation state that is ruined by the stress of travel,

    c) entering the home gives the experienced clinician/therapist much information regarding the patient and her relations to others and her material surroundings that can not be gathered in any other way, and

    d) the information thus gathered is instrumental in devising the next therapeutic thrust for the patient, especially in terms of the cognitive training. As described in various ways above, our treatment is highly individualized, although at the headline level it is the same for all MUS patients, i.e. cognitive training, relaxation and other therapies and medical advice, usually pertaining to reducing the number and amounts of medication the patient is on. Obviously, none of these activities can be planned or delivered in a standardized way, as each patient has her unique background, experience and reactions to the causing factors in MUS and to each session in the treatment;

3) Treatment is delivered by individuals uniquely qualified in their fields. The primary characteristic of the individual therapist is a can-do attitude toward the combination of psychological and somatic experiences the patient exhibits. All of our therapists have a great wealth of experience and breadth of knowledge. This is in contrast to the sub-specialty setting where a specific and highly focused knowledge is necessary. Although probably not the deciding factor of our success, the choice of personnel is an important factor. It is obvious to us that our qualifications are unique, but hardly unattainable. The who, what, when, where, how and why of this is another area in stark need of development;

4) Our treatment is individualized based on the primary exam and the development of the case – see example below for an illustration of this. Further, the flexibility of the treatment allows us to bring in relevant experts on an ad hoc basis generally with very short referral times, either because they are "in house" (have a service agreement with our clinic) or they are able to put our patients in between other demands on their time; and

5) *Back to work* is the output variable. All of our patients are victims of long-term sick leave and all have seriously wounded work mentality. The largest part of the therapy leading *back to work* is building resiliency that allows the chronic pain patient to master her pain sufficiently to let it go. The second largest part is to repair the wounded work mentality, and the third is to repair the surroundings of the patient keeping her in her straits. This includes the immediate family, the extended family where relevant and the work place when that comes to the fore. Again here, there is a huge and unmet need for developing personnel capable in assessing and massaging the workplace to accommodate the less than 100% fit.

Besides these 5 items we do one more thing for our patients when funding allows: we continue the therapeutic effort until success has been achieved (*back to work*), or until we are not able to move the patient forward. This is in contrast to most treatment modalities that are delivered based on specific criteria meting out measured therapeutic regimes (the more and more common DRG concept). We are of course limited by what the payer is willing to pay, yet we motivate continuation of treatment in cases where the average modality has given up. This is motivated by our experience that has shown that even in the most difficult cases, good results can be had when the long run is financed. This point is in our experience the most difficult for the uninitiated to fathom. No system any of us know (and they are many) offers the breadth and scope of what it takes to bring the MUS patient securely back to the work force. They all demonstrate various shortcomings that condition the chain breaking with undue consequences for the patient, that through these shortcomings experience yet another failure of the system to understand them and take them seriously. For every failure of the system to understand the MUS patient, the harder it is to reach them the next time around, in that the distrust fueled by system failure re-enforces the patient's perception that nothing can help them. We have numerous examples that qualify this which the reader is welcome to request if so desired.

The patients unable to re-enter (or enter) the workforce are "weaned" from our services cautiously, unless funding is suddenly revoked, which we have experienced more often than not. It is extremely important for the continued improvement of this group to give them a clear and candid picture of why they can not come back and how they can lead productive lives notwithstanding. This will often entail a protected work setting with a very limited number of work hours – 1 to 3 per day.

Treatment consists of a combination of therapies, including cognitive training led by a qualified psychologist, normally one visit per week but often more than that. The periodicity of this therapy is predicated by the need for the patient and her family to assimilate what transpired during the cognitive session, which always takes at least an hour and often up to two. Over the weeks, the patient becomes better attuned to the coupling between their emotional and psychological being and the concomitant bodily sensations, mostly pain related, that are tied to these. Obviously, this cannot be described in detail except at the individual patient level, since what actually transpires between the patient, her surroundings and the psychologist is highly variable and depends on individual characteristics, experience, resiliency pattern and emotional spectrum. The general strategy is to help the patient develop a clear picture of her response pattern to emotions and challenges in order to devise mastery tools that the patient can use to change her response pattern to a positive instead of negative pattern. Relaxation therapy supports this with various techniques described below. The patient is brought to more or less deep relaxation though these techniques, and this is a new sensation for most of our patients. They are used to being high strung, with little time during waking hours for themselves and even less time to relax and enjoy. Also these sessions are delivered in the home or nearby for the same reasons as for the cognitive therapy. As needed, other therapies are added ad hoc, the most common of which is physiotherapy. Our relaxation therapists supplant physiotherapists in many respects, but not in the general area of muscle strength training and movement evaluation and training. Other common additions to the therapeutic regime are mainly diagnostic and are usually referred in order to rule out serious disease when symptoms mimic those of such, e.g. serious chest and stomach pains or pains in joints or muscles that warrant further investigation. Such examinations are carried out in the public health care system, which in Denmark functions very well as long as the issue in question is clear and limited.

In our work, it is common that changes in the patient condition reveal other aspects of the case which further temper and guide the therapeutic process. Each case evolves individually, but one example will elucidate the value of this approach.

The patient in question has a minority religious belief and has grown up in a very restrictive environment under conditions conducive to the development of a dependent, escapist and externalizing personality. The woman in question is in her mid 30s and has two sons, both of which are bed-wetters at the ages of 9 and 12. The husband is the same age as the patient and works full time in a non-skilled position – he is of the same religious belief as the patient. The patient's presenting problem is a chronic fatigue syndrome with varying and severe pains. She has been described, as have nearly all of our patients, as having been through every imaginable specialist work-up, none of which have turned up anything clinically useful and/or of any help for the patient. Our first impression was of a patient with massive and mostly unconscious psychological mechanisms that are 1. closely related to her physical symptoms both temporally and in severity and 2. clearly predicating the physical symptoms the patient has. As professionals working in this field, it is clear that one cannot describe this diagnosis to the patient off hand – it would make it impossible to start therapy with most of the patients with these symptoms, as they would be angered and frustrated by being told that their symptoms are mostly if not wholly explainable by character traits and dysfunctional reaction patterns. In this specific case, the patient had been through a psychological treatment regime earlier and had been very put off by it.

Meanwhile, during the first few sessions, the patient began to thaw and it was demonstrable to her that the stresses in her daily routine had clear relationships to her symptoms. Although this was clear enough from the preliminary work-up, it took numerous psychologist sessions and guidance from the primary author to get the therapy on the right track, which included psychological tool building (cognitive training) around the dysfunctional reactions to improve the pattern. As the therapy was carried out in the patient's home, the relationships with her children and husband were evident and identifiable as elements in the problem complex. This underlines the value of the long-term treatment plan and the delivery mode in the patient's home.

We utilize relaxation therapists in our treatment. There is as yet no licensure scheme nor a clear professional identity of this group which is comprised of therapists of extremely variable quality. Therapists are evaluated by us based on previous experience and curriculum vitae. Only the best are accepted as members of our team.

This patient had, as most MUS patients have, a generally stressed muscle mass with special tenderness and tenseness of the back and neck muscles, giving rise to a nearly ubiquitous headache tendency, which among MUS patients is often misdiagnosed as migraine or Horton's headache (cluster headache). Relaxation therapy in our clinic is carried out by qualified therapists, who focus especially on the interface between psychological mechanisms and bodily function. Cranio-sacral therapy, somatic experiencing, acupuncture and music therapy are among the methods utilized. None of these are well documented in terms of specific therapeutic results, but all are continuously evaluated in house in terms of patient satisfaction, seminal improvement signs and interviews. The soft nature of this data is a necessary disadvantage when dealing with the MUS patient. No double blinded, controlled protocol would allow the therapeutic effort into the inner workings of the patient complex, and a sensitive and tolerant therapeutic effort is neither measurable nor standardizable.

As the therapy evolves, we evaluate from week to week if other therapies are indicated and instigate such as needed. Typical examples are warm water bathing/therapy with and without physiotherapeutic guidance, physiotherapy per se, consultations with other specialists, picture and/or laboratory diagnostic procedures and consultations with social and/or other authorities.

In the latter area, we make every effort to establish and/or reestablish the patient's work force related skills. This is carried out by specialized occupational consultants with a high degree of sensitivity to the problems the MUS patient has when returning to the work force, however light and easy the job may be. We spend considerable effort negotiating with the social authorities, who have the administrative and financial responsibility for optimizing the individual's work ability, but who rarely display understanding of the plight of the MUS patient. They rather have a prejudice regarding the MUS patient as being lazy or unacceptably socially dysfunctional and have a highly disconcerting record of doing more damage that good for the MUS patient (the primary author's own observations through 5 years of experience as a full-time medical consultant with 17 different municipal social services organizations). These negotiations and continued therapy during the re-socialization process (*back to work*) are central elements in our success rate.

Results

Based on 18 completed therapy regimens, 10 are back in the workforce or doing education with a clear work targeted output. Also here, no standardized approach is relevant – each patient and each case worker has to be individually treated. The important point here is to make the effort. It leads to results.

We have not yet been able to follow a sufficient number of patients to generalize concerning the applicability of the described treatment modality. However, the rationale and logic inherent in delivery of treatment in the patient's home, the interprofessional approach and the full spectrum of treatment delivery, from the intensive medical and psychotherapeutic intervention via less intensive therapy to therapeutically supported occupational training, are resoundingly clear.

Cost of Treatment

The treatment is expensive and highly demanding in therapy hours, but clearly worthwhile when over half of the patients thus treated return to the work force with all of the ramifications this has for the individual, her family, her community and society at large. Not investing in this endeavor is tantamount to writing a blank check to each MUS patient for life long disability pay. A rough estimate for the individual is as stated above approximately EUR 2,4 million, and a rough estimate of an average cost per treatment (including examination and the full spectrum of treatment including transport of staff) is EUR 35,000. It is not hard to figure the cost of doing nothing for MUS patients, which comprise approximately 3 percent of western societies, and other treatment modalities with worse than 50% success rates for *back to work* are saving that much less.

Conclusion

The described modality is dependent on qualified personnel. The field is in stark need of development, both of trained personnel as well as relevant financing models. There is a significant lack of understanding among medical personnel of the scope and breadth of the problem, and none less than awareness of what to do about it. Given that the described modality can be generalized and disseminated, there is no reason why at least half of the MUS disabled population can be brought back to the work force, resulting in enormous personal, professional and economic benefits.

It is clear that western societies have a serious and growing problem with that proportion of the population that does not fit the mold, is not able to function 100% under normal conditions. We are hurtling down the track with destination evidenced-based DRG. Unless we develop flexible and tolerant financing for effective treatment for MUS patients, we can not expect the cost of supporting them to come down. We have shown a way that works.

Literature

1 Koch H, van Bokhoven MA, Riet GT, van der Weijden T, Dinant GJ, Bindels PJ. Demographic characteristics and quality of life of patients with unexplained complaints: a descriptive study in general practice. Qual Life Res. 2007 Sep 26 (ahead of publication).

2 Fink P, Toft T, Hansen MS,Ombol E, Olesen F. Symptoms and syndromes of bodily distress: an exploratory study of 978 internal medical, neurological, and primary care patients. Psychosom Med. 2007 Jan;69(1):30-9.
3 Smith RC, Lyles JS, Gardiner JC, Sirbu C, Hodges A, Collins C, Dwamena FC, Lein C, William Given C, Given B, Goddeeris J. Primary care clinicians treat patients with medically unexplained symptoms: a randomized controlled trial. J Gen Intern Med. 2006 Jul;21(7):671-7.
4 Smith RC, Lein C, Collins C, Lyles JS, Given B, Dwamena FC, Coffey J, Hodges A, Gardiner JC, Goddeeris J, Given CW. Treating patients with medically unexplained symptoms in primary care. J Gen Intern Med. 2003 Jun;18(6):478-89. Review.
5 Goldberg D, Gask L, O'Dowd T. The treatment of somatization: Teaching techniques of reattribution. J Psychosom Research 1989; 33, 6: 698-695.
6 The healing circle: resiliency in nurses. Issues Ment Health Nurs. 2006 Jan;27(1):43-57. Review.
7 Feinstein AR. Clinimetrics. New Haven: Yale University Press, 1987.
8 Extensive discussions between the primary author and Dr. Feinstein prior to his demise.
9 Schmidt JG, Steele RE (eds), A Critical View of Medical Reasoning. Steps Toward a Timely Medical Practice: A Reader, Kircheim Press, Mainz, 1995.
10 Scaer RC. The Body Bears a Burden: Trauma, Dissociation and Disease, Haworth Press (USA) ISBN 0-7890-1245-6, 2001.
11 Cochrane, A.L. (1999) *Effectiveness and Efficiency: Random Reflections on Health Services*. The Royal Society of Medicine Press, London.
12 Rychetnik, L., P. Hawe, E. Waters, A. Barratt, & M. Frommer (2004) A glossary for evidence based public health. Journal of Epidemiology and Community Health, 58, 538-545.
13 Fink P, Rosendal M, Olesen F. Classification of somatization and functional somatic symptoms in primary care. Aust N Z J Psychiatry. 2004 Sep; 39(9):722-81.
14 Mackenbach JP, Borsboom GJ, Nusselder WJ, Looman CW, Schrivers CT. Determinants of levels and changes of physical functioning in chronically ill persons: results from the GLOBE study. J Epidemiol Community Health. 2001 Sep; 55(9): 631-8.
15 Bintzer M. Motor Conversion Disorder: Clinical characteristics and outcome among patients with medically unexplained loss of motor

function (doctoral disputation), self-published, Umeå 1998, ISBN 91-7191-518-4: 152pp. Doctoral disputation.
16 Valat JP, Goupille P, Védere V. Low back pain: risk factors for chronicity. Rev Rhum Engl Ed. 1997 Mar; 64(3):189-94. Review.
17 Fransen M, Woodward M, Norton R, Coggan C, Dawe M, Sheridan N. Risk factors associated with the transition from acute to chronic occupational back pain. Spine. 2002 Jan 1;27(1):92-8.
18 Press release, Danish Ministry of Social Affairs, May 31, 2006.
19 Healy D., Alfred G. Antidepressant drug use & the risk of suicide. Int Rev Psychiatry. 2005 Jun;17(3):163-72.
20 Rasmussen C. Hvis du skal bevise, du er syg, kan du ikke blive rask (translated: If you must prove you are ill, you cannot be cured). Medicus 2005; 5: 18-21.

CHAPTER THIRTEEN

ABOUT THE AUTHORS

http://www.paracelsus-heute.ch/cms/praxis/team/schmidt.php
Johannes G. Schmidt, specialist in General Medicine, Clinical Epidemiology (University of Newcastle/Australia), **Classical Chinese Medicine** (Master Hin Chung Got)

Johannes Schmidt was born in 1955 in Switzerland He attended primary school in Sirnach/Thurgau, and completed his medical education at the University of Basel, where he graduated in 1982. Between 1986 and 1987, he undertook his postgraduate studies of Clinical Epidemiology at the University of Newcastle/Australia, sponsored by the Swiss National Fund for Research (Nationalfonds). He did his MD thesis in 1990 at the University of Lausanne on the epidemiology of breast cancer screening in which he showed that mass mammography screening has no net benefit, but considerable harmful effects. He founded a clinic with several doctors, himself working as general practitioner with the use of the ancient classical Chinese medicine, i.e. acupuncture, herbal medicine and instructions on how to strengthen natural recovery. As a clinical epidemiologist, he is a specialist of evidence-based medicine. In practice, this resulted in therapies to help natural recovery with the use of mainly Chinese herbs and conventional medical therapies only where there is good evidence of a relevant benefit for the patient. Health should be achieved in a sustainable and lasting way. He has published scientific papers about screening, especially cancer screening, cholesterol screening and routine ultrasound in pregnancy. His analysis on the effects of breast cancer screening were published in the *Journal of Clinical Epidemiology* and had an effect on the international perception of the questionable benefit of breast cancer screening. He wrote the chapter about early detection and risk factor screening in the German textbook on General Medicine, edited by M Kochen. He was a member of the working group Preventive Medicine of the Federal committee on the appraisal of medical measures (Eidg. Leistungskommission). This work let him conclude that conventional medicine has no real concept for recovery and health vis a vis a health and resilience status that protects from further disease. At the end of 2016, he had to finish working because of health problems. Since 2018, he has lived in Thailand at his wife's farm, planting nice things such as coconuts, bananas, mangos, avocados, lemons, oranges and figs.

Richard Evan Steele, specialist in public health medicine and so much more, was born in 1952 on the shores of Lake Superior in Washburn, Wisconsin. He attended primary school in Wisconsin Rapids, Wisconsin and Ft. Collins, Colorado, and high school in Fort Collins. He spent much time in the mountains foraging and hunting/fishing, surviving during winter months in makeshift lean-to constructions, using bear claw snowshoes to move around in deep snow. He started school again after extensive travels on foot, cycling and motorcycling in all 48 continental United States, Alaska, all countries in Europe and most countries in Africa and the Middle East. His first post-secondary school degree was Laboratory Technical Bachelor of Science in 1980 from Aarhus Technical College. He studied medicine at Aarhus University 1980-1986. He ran more than 30 workshops during his medical studies on medical education and healthcare planning. He ran a workshop in 1988 for leading administrators of Odense University Hospital under the title of Odense University Hospital Year 2000. The group hatched the outline of a plan that later became the backbone of the strategy outlined in his book *Managed Care in a Public Setting* which boldly and practically describes the future of health care and social services. The workshop led to his being hired by the regional authority to put this plan into practice, but he soon realized that he did not have the tools or knowledge to make this happen. He therefore sought and obtained support from the Danish Research Academy to take a Master of Public Health and postdoctoral certificate in health services planning, international comparison and quality management at Johns Hopkins University. There he gained fame as a workshop guru and led the process for the CDC/HRSA Faculty/Agency Forum, which boldly and forcefully defined the much-needed collaboration between public health academe and public health practice. This led later to the establishment of the Washington, D.C. based Public Health Foundation and the Council on Linkages in Public Health. He is third on the author list of the *The Public Health Faculty/Agency: Linking Graduate Education and Practice: Final Report*. He is a board certified specialist in public health medicine and as is extremely unusual for this specialty has over 25 years of hands-on clinical experience in orthopedic surgery/acute medicine, cardiology, neurology and geriatrics, most at senior house level of expertise. He has authored and/or co-authored more than 30 publications including his autobiography, *Pushy? From Vagabond to Super Generalist Doctor: The Untold Story*. He has been a presenter/poster and author at dozens of international conferences. He is a John Maxwell trained coach, speaker and trainer. He lives in Sejs close to Silkeborg and celebrated the 47th anniversary of his marriage to his wife on February 6, 2023. He has 2 daughters, a son, and 6 grandchildren. He plays guitar, sings and dabbles a bit on the fiddle. He loves to cook and share a glass of wine at home. He runs a clinic with low level laser therapy and has successfully treated patients with whiplash syndrome, tension headache, post-concussion syndrome, asthma, chronic obstructive pulmonary disease, irritable bowel syndrome, eczema of all sorts, warts and many other inflammatory conditions.

Treat the patient, not the disease(s)